# Malaria in Africa

T0175214

# Challenges in Public Health

Editor: Prof. Dr. Oliver Razum, Bielefeld

Formerly/früher: Medizin in Entwicklungsländern
Herausgegeben von
Prof. Dr. Hans Jochen Diesfeld, Heidelberg

Band 60

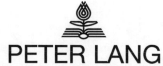

## PETER LANG

Frankfurt am Main · Berlin · Bern · Bruxelles · New York · Oxford · Wien

# Olaf Müller

# Malaria in Africa

## Challenges for Control and Elimination in the 21st Century

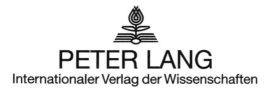

PETER LANG

Internationaler Verlag der Wissenschaften

**Bibliographic Information published by the Deutsche Nationalbibliothek**
The Deutsche Nationalbibliothek lists this publication in the Deutsche Nationalbibliografie; detailed bibliographic data is available in the internet at http://dnb.d-nb.de.

ISSN 1863-768X
ISBN 978-3-631-59792-7

© Peter Lang GmbH
Internationaler Verlag der Wissenschaften
Frankfurt am Main 2011
All rights reserved.

www.peterlang.de

# Table of contents

# Foreword

*"Malaria in Africa – challenges for control and elimination in the 21ˢᵗ century"* sticks out of the flood of malaria monographs after the latest edition of "Essential Malariology" by Leonard Bruce-Chwatt and his successors, Herbert M. Gilles and David A. Warrell (1993). A critical analysis of the past, an update leading to a visionary though critical outlook towards the future of malaria control and elimination is overdue.

Malaria is interacting with mankind and his evolution, ever since, until today, as Randall Packard (2008) argues. Malaria is the most ecologically sensitive of all human diseases. So have malaria parasites and vectors, men and their malariologists mutually influenced each other in terms of strategies and anti-strategies. The first science-based – or should one say accidental breakthrough in modern malariology was a new vector control tool, DDT, in the 1940s. This added to the so far mainly indirect, ecological and socio-economic tools to control malaria. Between 1955 and 1969 most of malaria-endemic regions in Europe, the Americas and partly Asia could rid themselves, with the World Health Organisation (WHO) and international assistance, from this dreadful burden, whereby a positive interaction between disease control and socio-economic development cannot be denied. The looser at that time was and still is Africa. After that initial success story came a period of depression, complacency, development of resistance of parasites and vectors against chemicals, and most importantly, a waning political and academic interest. Packards ironically commented: "DDT did not eliminate malaria, only malariologists".

Africa remained the home of the most aggressive malaria parasite, *P. falciparum*, and the most effective vector species, *An. gambiae*, in the ecologically most favourable and socio-economically and politically most instable environment. Malaria is adding to the vicious cycle of poverty and disease. Some 50 years after the introduction of DDT, in 1997 a new effort was started by the international scientific and donor community to attack malaria once more. Modern biosciences detected plasmodia as a new field of interest thus giving new impetus to fundamental and applied parasitological, entomological, genetic and clinical research leading to new insights into the complex phenomenon of malaria. Backed by an unprecedented international political and financial will and supported by public-private foundations, new initiatives were started with new goals and targets. In spite of all these efforts over the past 15 years, still a million

7

malaria deaths occur every year, 90% of it in tropical Africa, where only 10% of the world's population live.

Therefore Africa is the focus of this book. The great advantage of it is that malaria is put in a holistic context, which enables the young reader who wants to familiarise him/herself with the problem of malaria comprehensively. The natural history of the disease is put into the context of political, economic, ecological but also of researchers, international organizations and health policy driven-interests, who determine the input, output and outcome of malaria control efforts. The old, almost ancient dilemma: vertical versus horizontal approach; bio-scientific versus socio-economic, political and ecological approach is being discussed. The most important message is the statement that with all the presently available knowledge and tools malaria could come under control also in Africa, if only the political will at national and international level would strengthen the overall health system in the context of true Primary Health Care (PHC) and if PHC would be taken seriously as a tool to reach the Millennium Development Goals (MDG). Here scepticism is more than justified.

The author whose 20 years of malaria research in Africa are truly the basis of this comprehensive update and reader is to be congratulated to this thoughtful and critical account of a still highly relevant human health problem.

*Starnberg, November 2010*

*Hans-Jochen Diesfeld*

# Preface

It is now about 25 years ago that I had started to work on aspects of public health in tropical Africa. In 1985, I became a doctoral student of the *Berlin School of Tropical Medicine* and I was sent for a period of six months to the small town of Manono in the eastern part of former Zaire. In this very remote and poor community, I learned my first and intense lessons about malaria and other tropical diseases and their associations with poverty. While conducting specific field work on aspects of hepatomegaly and schistosomiasis at the local hospital and in the surrounding villages, I already realised the major impact of malaria on morbidity and mortality in such poor communities.

In the following years while undergoing clinical and public health training in Germany, I worked particularly in the field of HIV/AIDS control in sub-Saharan Africa (SSA). Having been responsible for projects supported by non-governmental organisations (NGOs) in Uganda and the *German Technical Cooperation* (GTZ) in Zaire, I was able to conduct a number of studies on the associations between malaria and HIV/AIDS in patients of local hospitals. In addition, I did consultancies on GTZ-supported disease control projects in other malaria-endemic countries of central and eastern Africa.

Upon completion of my specialisation in public health in Europe, I had the opportunity to work as a malaria epidemiologist and served as the head of the Farafenni field station of the *British Medical Research Council* (MRC) laboratories in The Gambia. This intense experience at the largest tropical medicine research institution at that time in SSA, which had a clear focus on malaria research, has influenced me greatly. I will never forget the rainy season of the year 1995, when I spent much of my time in the MRC Farafenni outpatient clinic having been responsible for the routine services and the conduct of clinical malaria studies. The number of desperate mothers arriving with their seriously ill children, who mostly had full blown cerebral malaria, increased steadily with the onset of malaria transmission, and many of these children died despite rapid and correct treatment provision. Here, I became really aware what is meant by malaria as the "killer disease" of young African children. During my work at the MRC in The Gambia I also learned more about the value of applied research through my involvement in various epidemiological studies, for example in the evaluation of the *Gambian National Impregnated Bed Net Program*, the first of its kind in SSA.

Since 1997 I am working at the *Institute of Public Health* (formerly *Department of Tropical Hygiene and Public Health)* at the Heidelberg University, where I am teaching *Strategies and Policies of Disease Control* besides conducting applied research on the control of tropical infectious diseases in Africa. In close collaboration with a well established national research institute, the *Nouna Health Research Centre,* and with funding from the *Deutsche Forschungsgemeinschaft* (DFG) in the framework of the specific research programme (Sonderforschungsbereich) *"Control of Tropical Infectious Diseases"* (SFB 544), I was responsible for numerous epidemiological, clinical and public health oriented research projects in this highly malaria endemic area of north-western Burkina Faso. The results of this research have further opened my eyes for the devastating effects of malaria in SSA communities and have finally motivated me to write this book.

*Heidelberg, December 2010*

*Olaf Müller*

# List of abbreviations

| | |
|---|---|
| ACPR | Adequate Clinical and Parasitological Response |
| ACT | Artemisinin-based Combination Therapy |
| AMFm | Affordable Medicines Facility for Malaria |
| ANC | Antenatal care |
| ART | Antiretroviral drug Treatment |
| BCE | Before the Common Era |
| BS | *Bacillus sphaericus* |
| BTI | *Bacillus thueringensis israelensis* |
| CDC | U.S. Centers for Disease Control and Prevention |
| CRSN | Centre de Recherche en Santé de Nouna |
| DALY | Disability-Adjusted Life Year |
| DDT | Dichlorodiphenyl-trichlorethane |
| DFG | Deutsche Forschungsgemeinschaft |
| DFID | Department for International Development |
| DHS | Demographic and Health Surveys |
| DNDi | Drugs against Neglected Diseases Initiative |
| DPT | Diphtheria, Pertussis and Tetanus |
| DSS | Demographic Surveillance System |
| EIR | Entomological Inoculation Rate |
| EPI | Extended Programme of Immunization |
| ETF | Early Treatment Failure |
| FAO | United Nations Food and Agriculture Organization |
| G6PD | Glucose-6-phosphate dehydrogenase |
| GAVI | Global Alliance for Vaccines and Immunization |
| GDP | Gross Domestic Product |
| GHI | Global Health Initiatives |
| GMAP | Global Malaria Action Plan |
| GSK | GlaxoSmithKline |
| GTZ | German Technical Cooperation |
| HCH | Hexachlorocyclohexane |
| HDSS | Health and Demographic Surveillance System |
| HIS | Health information system |
| IEC | Information/Education/Communication |
| IMF | International Monetary Fund |

| | |
|---|---|
| INDEPTH | *International Network for the Demographic Evaluation of Populations and Their Health in developing countries* |
| IPT | Intermittent Preventive Treatment |
| IPTc | Intermittent Preventive Treatment in young children |
| IPTi | Intermittent Preventive Treatment in infants |
| IPTp | Intermittent Preventive Treatment in pregnant women |
| IRS | Indoor insecticide Residual Spraying |
| ITM | Insecticide-Treated Material |
| ITN | Insecticide-Treated Mosquito Net |
| IVCC | Innovative Vector Control Consortium |
| LCF | Late Clinical Failure |
| LDC | Least Developed Countries |
| LLIN | Long-Lasting Insecticidal Nets |
| LPF | Late Parasitological Failure |
| MDA | Mass Drug Administration |
| MDG | Millennium Development Goals |
| MEG | Malaria Elimination Group |
| MIM | Multilateral Initiative on Malaria |
| MMV | Medicines for Malaria Venture |
| MRC | British Medical Research Council |
| MRL | Maximum Residual Limit |
| MVI | Malaria Vaccine Initiative |
| NGO | Non-Governmental Organisation |
| OECD | Organisation of Economic Co-operation and Development |
| PAHO | Pan American Health Organisation |
| PCR | Polymerase Chain Reaction |
| PDP | Product Development Partnerships |
| PEM | Protein Energy Malnutrition |
| PHC | Primary Health Care |
| PMI | The US President's Malaria Initiative |
| POP | Persistent Organic Pollutant |
| PPP | Public-Private Partnerships |
| RBM | Roll Back Malaria Initiative |
| RCT | Randomised Controlled Trial |
| RDT | Rapid Diagnostic Test |
| SFB | Sonderforschungsbereich (Specific Research Programme) |
| SSA | Sub-Saharan Africa |
| UNDP | United Nations Development Programme |
| UNICEF | United Nations International Children's Emergency Fund |
| USAID | U.S. Agency for International Development |

| | |
|---|---|
| VHW | Village Health Workers |
| WB | World Bank |
| WHO | World Health Organisation |
| WHOPES | WHO Pesticides Evaluation Scheme |
| WHO-TDR | WHO Special Programme for Research and Training in Tropical Diseases |

# Introduction

In 1994, some 2.300 million people (41% of the world population) from 100 countries and territories were living in regions of malaria endemicity. The global incidence of malaria at that time was estimated at 300-500 million clinical cases annually, causing between 1.5-2.7 million deaths each year (WHO 1997). A decade later, the situation had not changed much, with still roughly half of the world's population in 107 countries having been at risk for the disease (Breman et al. 2006) (figure 1). Global malaria morbidity at that time was estimated to be still half a billion clinical cases per year, causing between one and three million deaths (Greenwood et al. 2005, Breman et al. 2006, WHO 2009b). With the successes of the *Roll Back Malaria Initiative* (RBM), the global malaria burden has now started to decrease significantly (WHO 2009b). However, it is difficult to measure malaria morbidity and mortality, as the clinical symptoms are rather unspecific and as most of the deaths in malaria endemic regions occur at home without any report from health workers (Müller 2000). Malaria thus remains among the leading causes of global morbidity and mortality and is certainly the most important parasitic disease of humans (Greenwood et al. 2005).

At the beginning of the $21^{st}$ century, the great majority of the malaria burden falls on the poor rural communities in sub-Saharan Africa (SSA) and most deaths occur in young children (Greenwood et al. 1987, Snow et al. 2005, Müller et al. 2003) (figure 1). Malaria in pregnancy is also a major cause of severe maternal anaemia and low birth-weight babies, which contributes significantly to maternal and infant mortality (Greenwood et al. 2005). Of the 107 countries in which malaria remains endemic, 45 are within the WHO African region (WHO 2009b). Malaria has rightly been considered to be a major barrier to the development of SSA (Sachs & Malaney 2002), as well as an indicator for the persistence of global structural inequality (Stratton et al. 2008).

After a failed *Global Malaria Eradication Campaign* – which was not truly global as it has left out the entire African continent – spanning from 1955 until 1969 and being followed by a long period of neglect, malaria has received renewed interest and support since the 1990s (Müller 2000, Müller 2006). This development started with a meeting of African health ministers in Dakar/Senegal in 1992 and has paved the way to the establishment of RBM, a successful global partnership with its secretariat at WHO headquarter in Geneva (Nabarro & Taylor 1998, Müller 2006). Since then and particularly in the past five years there has been

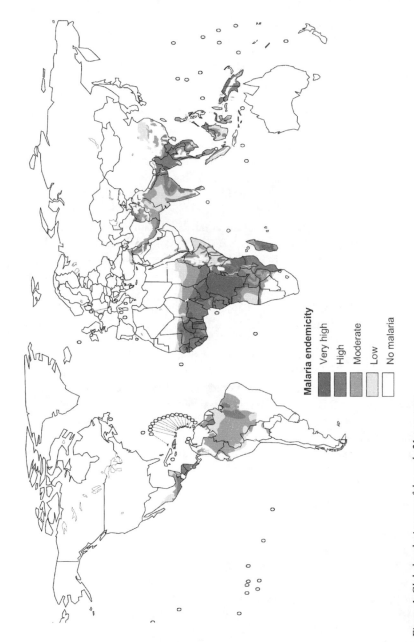

Figure 1: Global malaria map of the early 21st century
Source: WHO (2005)

Malaria endemicity

- Very high
- High
- Moderate
- Low
- No malaria

a major increase in global funding for malaria research and control through new international initiatives such as the *Global Fund to fight HIV/AIDS, Tuberculosis and Malaria* (Global Fund), the US *President's Malaria Initiative* (PMI) and the *World Bank's Booster Programme*, but also through numerous activities of NGOs and other public-private partnerships (Müller 2006, WHO 2008b, Mendis et al. 2009).

It was in October 2007 at a meeting of the *Bill and Melinda Gates Foundation* (Gates Foundation) in Seattle/USA that the term malaria eradication (eradication = reduction to zero of the incidence in the whole world) was introduced again into the international discussion (Okie 2008). Since then, the feasibility of global malaria eradication continues to be hotly debated (Feachem &Sabot 2008, Tanner & de Savigny 2008, Greenwood et al. 2008, Mendis et al. 2009). However, it should be remembered that the situation in 1955 resembled very much the situation today. The decision to launch a global eradication effort was at that time much influenced by the availability of two very effective tools, firstly and primarily the insecticide dichlorodiphenyl-trichlorethane (DDT) and secondly the antimalarial drug chloroquine (Müller 2000). Today, we again rely on only two and for the time being very effective tools, insecticide-treated mosquito nets (ITNs) and artemisinin-based combination therapies (ACT) (Greenwood et al. 2008). This has now led to the development of the very detailed *Global Malaria Action Plan* of the RBM initiative which emphasises the final goal of malaria eradication (RBM 2008).

However, we need to remember that it was not only the development of resistance of the malaria vectors to DDT and its costly successors and the development of resistance of the malaria parasites against chloroquine and the following monotherapies that led to the principal failure of the *Global Malaria Eradication Campaign* of the last century, but the mistake to not fully take into account the overall weakness of the national health systems in the tropical regions of Asia and Latin America at that time (Müller 2000). In particular, the vertical structure of the national malaria elimination (elimination = reduction to zero of the incidence in a defined geographical area) programmes in respective endemic countries prevented early successes to be sustained. As a consequence, malaria globally resurged even in tropical countries where it was nearly eliminated (Müller 2000). Today, there is an obvious risk to simply repeat such mistakes of the past, if the RBM continues to invest in tools development and provision without systematically and massively strengthening the health systems of SSA countries (Müller 2000, Greenwood et al. 2008). Moreover, it is important to note that the epidemiology of malaria in SSA is quite different from malaria in other regions of the world (Snow et al. 2005). Thus the malaria community needs a thorough discussion regarding which strategies should be used and how much could realistically be achieved with the existing tools under the real life conditions in SSA today.

This book aims to provide a comprehensive update on the recent developments of the epidemiology of malaria and existing strategies and tools for malaria control and elimination in Africa. It discusses recent developments and plans in the context of the long global history of malaria control and points to the many challenges the RBM faces today on the African continent. The book aims to address a wide audience, from master and doctoral students interested in global health issues, over basic, clinical and social scientists working on research in the field of malaria and tropical diseases, to public health practitioners engaged in health and development projects and programmes of malaria endemic countries in Africa.

# Chapter 1. Global history of malaria

## 1.1 Ancient history

Modern humankind gradually developed in tropical Africa over the last 300.000 years. The dominating malaria parasites of humans are likely to originate from Africa, where remarkably similar parasites of man and primates exist (Bruce-Chwatt 1988). The hypothesis of a long co-evolution is furthermore supported by the fact that the malaria parasites of primates only develop in *Anopheles* mosquitoes (Bruce-Chwatt 1988). During much of the years of development of *Homo sapiens* in Africa, malaria must have been a restricted zoonosis in self-containing small foci (Webb 2009a). Such endemic foci probably occurred in small human settlements on riverbanks and in areas of cleared rainforest in tropical Africa, long before the first major riverine civilizations of humankind became established (Webb 2009a). Thus, the prehistoric emergence of malaria as an endemic disease had already taken place when human populations first transitioned from hunting and food-gathering societies to food-producing societies, which are a requirement for successful transmission of any communicable disease (Webb 2009a). Moreover, the clearing of rain forests together with the high prevalence of tsetse flies, which prevented humans to keep livestock in many areas of SSA, were fundamental for the development of the marked anthropophily and thus outstanding transmission capacity of *Anopheles gambiae* and *Anopheles funestus*, the two principal malaria vectors on this continent (Webb 2009a).

Genetic evidence points to *Plasmodium vivax* being probably two to three million years old, but where and how it developed in Africa is not fully understood (Webb 2009a). It is likely that vivax malaria has accompanied humankind over a period of tens of thousands of years in parallel to the process of the human cultural evolution in SSA. The early patterns of riverbank settlement, rainforest cultivation and seasonal migration might have provided ideal conditions for seasonal transmission of *P. vivax*, due to its potential for relapse of infections (Webb 2009a). However, this co-evolution over time has also enabled African populations to develop a nearly perfect protection from this parasite by selecting for Red Blood Cell Duffy antigen negativity. Today, some 97 percent of the West and Central African populations carry the mutation for Duffy negativity (Webb 2009a).

It is not very clear how the modern form of *Plasmodium falciparum* developed, but genetic evidence points to the emergence of human infections during the period 13,000 to 8,000 BCE and thus significantly later than *P. vivax* (Webb 2009a). Latest research on this topic makes it likely that *P. falciparum* originates from a similar parasite which infects the African gorilla and which is now called *gorilla P. falciparum* (Liu et al. 2010). Such a time-line is also reflected by the relatively young association between *P. falciparum* and the sickle cell (HbS) gene. Although HbS homozygotes are experiencing high mortality, HbS heterozygotes are much less susceptible for falciparum malaria and thus have a survival advantage. Such a balanced HbS polymorphism is regularly seen in regions where *P. falciparum* was or is highly endemic, including SSA (Hill 1992). Moreover, the transmission dynamics of *P. falciparum* require a stable relationship between large human populations and mosquito vectors, which only seems possible during the later phases of human cultural evolution.

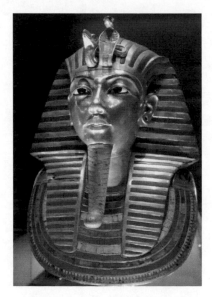

*Figure 2: King Tutankhamen from Egypt, who died in 1324 B.C. at age 18 of malaria*
*Source: Wikipedia; www.wikipedia.org/wiki/Tutankhamun, accessed 13.10.2010*

The clinical and epidemiological features of malaria facilitated the historical differentiation of this disease from other clinical events. Earliest reports of seasonal and intermittent fevers date back several thousand years, and the clinical signs and symptoms of malaria were already reported in documents from the advanced civilizations of Mesopotamia, India, China, Greece and Egypt (Bruce-Chwatt 1988, Hawass et al. 2010) (figure 2). The *Artemesia* plant was used in China some 2000 years ago against fevers resembling malaria (White 2008) (figure 3). As mentioned before, malaria has accompanied man since prehistoric times in Africa. In more recent times, malaria was known to be very common in the southern valley of the Nile but not so much in northern Egypt. About 3,000 years old mummies with enlarged spleens were found, and a disease with fever and splenomegaly is mentioned in the Ebers Papyrus of 1,570 BCE (Bruce-Chwatt 1988). During the history of European exploration and exploitation, the African coast was known as "the white man's grave", with reported annual mortality rates of 54 per thousand among staff of the Royal Navy and even much greater losses during expeditions to discover the courses of the Niger and the Congo rivers (Bruce-Chwatt 1988). Malaria, beside yellow fever and other infectious diseases, must have had a great share on this burden.

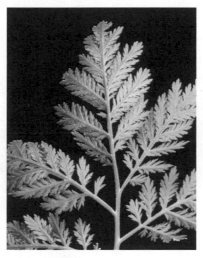

*Figure 3: Artemesia annua (annual wormwood)*
*Source: Anonymous (2005)*

In the early 17th century, the South-American Cinchona tree was revealed to be efficacious against malaria fevers (figure 4). However, it took quite some time, lots of controversies and expeditions of Alexander von Humboldt and others before this new remedy gradually got accepted as useful against malaria fevers (Bruce-Chwatt 1988). In the 19th century, the crews of the Royal Navy off the coast of West Africa were already systematically protected from malaria through quinine prophylaxis (Bruce-Chwatt 1988). Quinine prophylaxis for the indigenous African populations was rather an exemption than the rule, but was advocated by Robert Koch and partly used in German colonies (Clyde 1962, Bruce-Chwatt 1988). From the product of the bark of this tree, which was later called „Jesuit's Powder", the active substance quinine was isolated in 1820 in France (Gilles 1993).

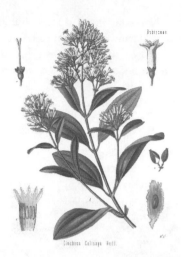

*Figure 4: Cinchona tree*
*Source: Wikipedia; www.wikipedia.org/wiki/Cinchona, accessed 07.11.2010*

The theory that poisonous air from swamps causes malaria dates back to ancient Greece. During the 17th and 18th centuries, there was the common belief that intermittent fevers were caused by the foul air in marshy areas and that this miasma entered the body by inhalation (Poser & Bruyn 1999). This led to the name *mal'aria* (bad air) in the Italian Peninsula, where this term was first used in the year 1560 (Bruce-Chwatt 1988). However, an association between mosquitoes and malaria fevers was suspected in many countries and cultures (Poser & Bruyn 1999). In northern Tanzania for example, malaria was attributed to mosquitoes from lowland areas which were known to be absent in highland areas, and this was reflected by the use of similar local names for mosquitoes and malaria, *m'bu* and *M'bu* respectively (Clyde 1962).

Malaria has become a predominantly tropical disease only in the very recent history of humankind (figure 5). Before the 20th century, malaria was prevalent on all continents and in nearly all countries of the world (Poser & Bruyn 1999). It was thus also a major problem in the whole of Europe, where it took a great toll over the years, particularly in southern Europe. In Italy the impact of the disease was well documented. A staggering number of popes had died of a fever which was most likely to be due to malaria, during the last centuries and some 15,000 deaths were reported annually in late 19th century from this country (Poser & Bruyn 1999, Dopson 1999). Malaria was also a large problem on the whole American continent. Although it is not entirely clear how the malaria parasites reached the Americas, there is evidence that this was through the Spanish conquerors and their African slaves (Poser & Bruyn 1999).

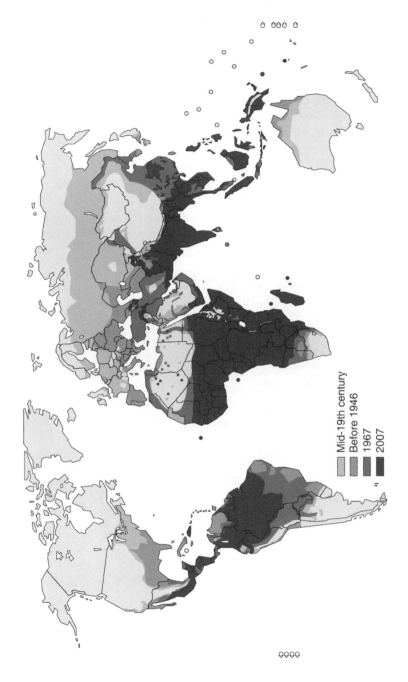

Figure 5: *Geographical distribution of malaria from 1900 until 2002*
*Source: Mendis et al. (2009)*

Mid-19th century
Before 1946
1967
2007

## 1.2 Discovery of the *Plasmodium* lifecycle (1880-1948)

The discovery of the malaria parasite through the French army physician Charles Laveran on November 6th 1880 in Algeria, who in fact saw the gametocytes of *P. falciparum* in the blood of a patient, was a major breakthrough in medical history (Poser & Bruyn 1999) (figure 6). This important discovery, which was awarded with the Nobel Prize in 1907, was however preceded by invaluable work of many more scientists in this field (Bruce-Chwatt 1988). Laveran's findings were confirmed later in Italy by Angelo Celli and colleagues, and it was again the Italian scientists who first described in detail the morphology and the clinical characteristics of the main human malaria parasites *P. falciparum, P. vivax* and *P. malariae* (Dopson 1999). It took however quite some time and many controversial discussions and publications before the discovery of Laveran was finally accepted by the leading scientists of his epoque (Poser & Bruyn 1999). The liver stages of the malaria parasites of man only got described three decades later (figure 7).

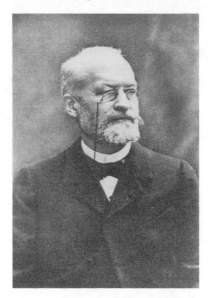

*Figure 6: Alphonse Laveran*
*Source: Wikipedia; www.wikipedia.org/wiki/AlphonseLavaran, accessed 07.11.2010*

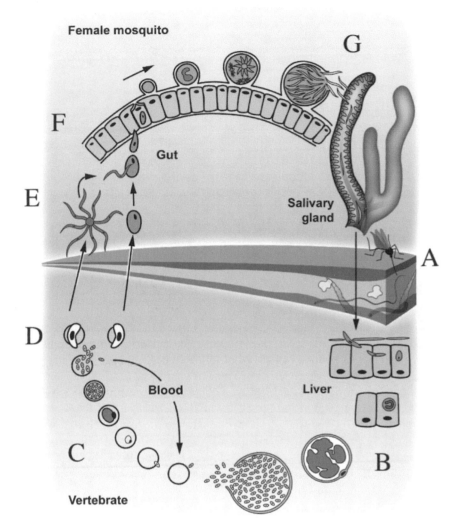

*Figure 7: The life cycle of malaria species in humans.*
Plasmodium *sporozoites enter a human host during the bite of an* Anopheles *mosquito (A). They reach the liver via the blood stream and multiply into thousands of merozoites (B). Merozoites enter the blood circulation and invade erythrocytes where they replicate and invade further erythrocytes (C). Some merozoites develop to gametocytes (D), which are subsequently taken up by an* Anopheles *mosquito (E). In the mosquito, a zygote develops which becomes an ookinete penetrating the midgut epithelium (F). The resulting oocysts generate the sporozoites which enter the mammalian host via the salivary glands (G).*
*Source: Courtesy Friedrich Frischknecht*

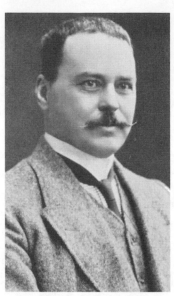

*Figure 8: Ronald Ross*
*Source: Wikipedia; www.wikipedia.org/wiki/RonaldRoss, accessed 07.11.2010*

Although the mosquito-malaria hypothesis was stated by many scientists including Laveran before, the natural transmission of the malaria parasite remained a mystery until the 20th of August 1897 in India, when the British army physician Ronald Ross – guided by the "father of Tropical Medicine", Patrick Manson – described the full mosquito-malaria life cycle in birds (Bruce-Chwatt 1988) (figure 8). Within a year, the complete life cycles of *P. falciparum* and *P. vivax* in the human and in the vector were described by Giovanni Battista Grassi and colleagues in Italy, including a successful transmission experiment with a volunteer bitten by malaria-infected *Anopheles* mosquitoes (Dopson 1999). In 1900, Patrick Manson himself conducted two very convincing experiments which proved again the transmission of human malaria by infected *Anopheles* mosquitoes. The first experiment was the exposure of volunteers to malaria in a highly endemic area in Italy, where they remained for a couple of months every night from sunset until one hour after sunrise in a mosquito-proof hut, without acquiring malaria. This confirmed similar experiments conducted by Grassi and colleagues in the same year (Dopson 1999). The second experiment was the transport of *Anopheles* mosquitoes that had fed on malaria cases in Italy to London, where they were allowed to bite two volunteers (one of them being Manson's son), both of whom developed tertian malaria afterwards (Poser & Bruyn 1999). Quite controversially, it was only Ronald Ross who was awarded the Nobel Prize in 1902 (Bruce-

Chwatt 1988). This was followed by a long and bitter rivalry between Ross and Grassi in which all the leading European scientists were involved (Poser & Bruyn 1999). This tragic story resembles a similar controversy in recent years, when the two scientists Luc Montagnier from France and Robert Gallo from the USA both claimed the discovery of the viral cause of AIDS, but only Montagnier got awarded the Nobel Prize in 2008 (Anonymous 2008a).

## 1.3 Drugs, insecticides and first success stories (1900-1930)

With the discovery of the origin of the disease, rational malaria control measures were rapidly implemented and there was optimism that malaria would soon become much reduced globally (Gilles 1993). In 1899 in Sierra Leone, Ronald Ross himself started a project based on larviciding with mineral oil, which showed some success but was not sustained (Bruce-Chwatt 1988).

In Tanzania and with the beginning of the 20th century, quinine began to slowly replace fever treatment with alcoholic beverages and mass treatment with quinine was subsequently introduced in the capital of the country, Dar es Salaam (Clyde 1962). Strongly influenced by Robert Koch, who had visited Tanzania first in 1898, and who – in opposition to the British school – preferred controlling malaria through a drug-based as against a vector control-based approach in addition to personal protection (e.g. with mosquito nets), mass treatment with quinine for all microscopically confirmed malaria cases and carriers started in the highly endemic city of Dar es Salaam already in 1901 (Clyde 1962). Although the dosage of quinine for this purpose was still controversial, the campaign was considered a success and was sustained until the beginning of World War I in 1914. Afterwards, malaria control continued in Tanzania but with not so well-coordinated vector control activities through drainage and/or application of weekly mineral oil or Paris Green mixed with gravel in breeding places (Clyde 1962). In 1926, broader access to quinine by placing the drug on sale at cost prize in post offices throughout the country was increasingly achieved. This system of drug distribution continued for the next 30 years in Tanzania, but quinine became later replaced by mepacrine and then finally by chloroquine (Clyde 1962). After World War II, indoor insecticide residual spraying (IRS) with DDT was first used in houses in Dar es Salaam and later also from airplanes. Malaria control operations got coordinated at that time by the Ross Institute of London under the supervision of George McDonald (Clyde 1962).

In the early 20th century, the Pan American Health Organisation (PAHO) recommended to its member governments the widespread distribution of information on malaria, the free distribution of quinine to the poor and the exemption from taxation of all products used in the prevention and treatment of this disease (Najera 1989, Najera 2001). The great success of the malaria (and yellow fever) control efforts of General William Crawford Gorgas in Cuba and Panama were based on the systematic employment of larvicides like Paris Green or simple mineral oils (Harrison 1978). There were many more or less successful malaria control projects during the first quarter of the 20th century in several malaria endemic countries including some African countries (e.g. Algeria, Egypt, Sudan, South Africa) (Bruce-Chwatt 1988, Mabaso et al. 2004). However, control of mosquito larvae through draining and oiling procedures as well as through larvivorous fish in ponds, control of adult mosquitoes through application of natural pyrethroids, and reduction of man-vector contact through mosquito-proofing of houses and bed netting proved to be too complicated and costly for large-scale application in large rural tropical regions (Gramiccia & Beales 1988). During the first half of the 20th century, effective malaria control in poor countries was thus largely restricted to certain urban areas and to specific communities, such as military and key industrial and agricultural areas (Harrison 1978).

In the northern countries of Europe as well as in the USA, indigenous malaria receded by the middle of the 19th century, due to a combination of environmental interventions (e.g. drainage, reclamation of coastal land), agricultural developments (e.g. increase in the number of cattle which deviated the zoophilic vectors from man to cattle), greater availability of quinine, and overall socioeconomic development (e.g. better housing, improved water supply). In the 20th century, malaria was more of a problem in southern Europe, where intense malaria control measures consequently became widely employed, particularly in the Mediterranean countries. In Italy, two different malaria control philosophies were battling each other. The first opinion was initiated by Battista Grassi and was represented by Angelo Celli, who emphasised that malaria is primarily a disease of poverty and who successfully lobbied for governmental distribution of affordable quinine together with the concept of *bonification* (reclamation of marshland, limitation of land ownership and resettlement of populations) (Gramiccia & Beales 1988). The second opinion was initiated by Ronald Ross and was supported by the Rockefeller Foundation, emphasizing primarily a vector control approach. With the assistance of the Rockefeller Foundation, vector control measures were key in successful elimination of the accidental invasions of *Anopheles gambiae* in Brazil in 1940 and in Egypt in 1945 as well as for the elimination of malaria from Cyprus, and this largely influenced further developments (Bruce-Chwatt 1988).

The development of modern synthetic drugs against malaria began with the detection of the antimalarial efficacy of the aniline dye methylene blue at the end of the 19th century (Guttmann & Ehrlich 1891). The dramatic experiences with malaria during World War I –when malaria already caused more deaths than the fighting activities on the battle fields – stimulated the development of synthetic antimalarial drugs in Germany, resulting in the detection of pamaquine (Plasmochin) in 1924, mepacrine (Atebrin) in 1930 and chloroquine (Resorchin) in 1934. Further milestones in the development of synthetic antimalarial drugs were the detection of proguanil in 1944, primaquine in 1950, and pyrimethamine in 1952 in France, the USA and the UK respectively (Müller 2000). By that time it appeared as if the arsenal of antimalarial drugs was almost complete with the availability of effective drugs against all stages of the parasite (Gramiccia & Beales 1988). The large-scale application of chloroquine started only after World War II, but a few years later it had already become the drug of choice for the treatment of nearly all uncomplicated malaria attacks worldwide (Gilles 1993) (figure 9).

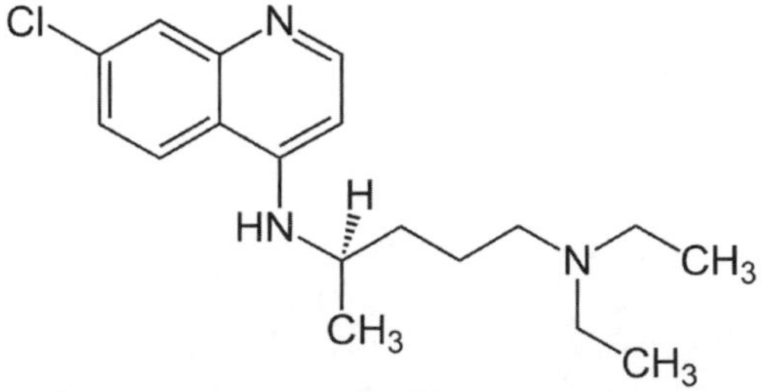

Figure 9: Chloroquine molecule
Source: Wikipedia; www.wikipedia.org/wiki/chloroquine, accessed 13.10.2010

The discovery of synthetic antimalarial drugs in the 20th century was paralleled by the development of insecticides against *Anopheles* mosquitoes. The successful application of natural pyrethroids in China, India and South Africa documented for the first time the effectiveness of malaria control strategies based on vector control (Bruce-Chwatt 1988, Mabaso et al. 2004). However, despite large-scale production of plant-based pyrethrum powder in many countries including Kenya and the former Belgian-Congo, weekly spraying programmes were considered unrealistic for tropical countries due to logistics and costs. During World War II, the high insecticidal action of DDT (figure 10) – which was first synthesized in Germany in 1874 – was demonstrated by Paul Müller in Switzerland in 1939, who was awarded the Nobel Prize for this discovery in 1948 (Poser & Bruyn 1999). This compound proved to be easily manufactured, to persist for a long time on sprayed surfaces, to effectively kill insects by simple contact, and to have a low toxicity to man (Harrison 1978). First successful field tests with DDT were carried out in Italy in collaboration with the Rockefeller Foundation in 1943, and the value of this insecticide for the interruption of malaria transmission was subsequently confirmed through its successful large-scale application in countries like Venezuela, Guyana, Ceylon, USA, Italy and Greece (Gilles 1993). Successful IRS programmes based on DDT also got established already by the 1940th in a number of southern African countries (Mabaso et al. 2004).

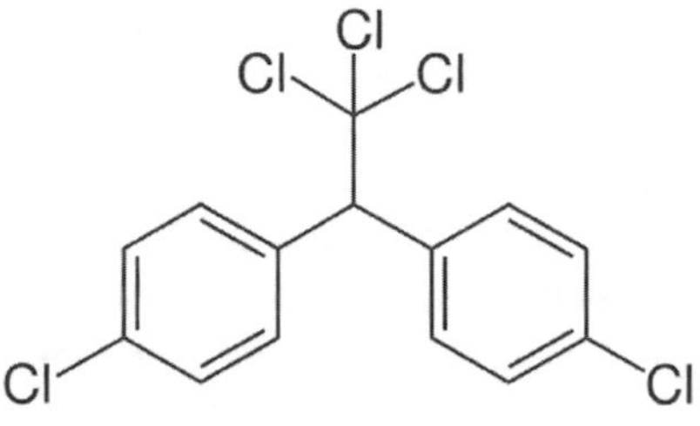

*Figure 10: DDT molecule*
*Source: Wikipedia; www.wikipedia.org/wiki/DDT, accessed 20.09.2010*

After World War II, the newly established WHO promised to devote more attention to the health needs of developing tropical regions and in particular to the enormous social and economic damage that malaria caused to the affected countries (Harrison 1978). As a consequence, the Interim Commission of WHO convened an *Expert Committee on Malaria* which met for the first time in 1947 to discuss the feasibility of global malaria eradication (Bruce-Chwatt 1988). The Committee made recommendations to the *First World Health Assembly* in 1948, which included the establishment of malaria control demonstration teams in endemic countries composed of a malariologist, an entomologist and a sanitarian together with national members. These teams tried to investigate the feasibility and the outcomes of locally adapted malaria control interventions, particularly DDT spraying operations (Gramiccia & Beales 1988). The number of demonstration teams in operation increased from 10 in 1950 to 35 in 1953. Over the period 1944-56, DDT was tried for malaria control in pilot projects or programmes in more than 120 countries, 46 having been situated in Africa (Gramiccia & Beales 1988). Already at that time, limited resistance of certain malaria vectors to DDT and alternative insecticides was observed, as well as the fact that the rapidly increasing insecticide resistance of other nuisance insects such as flies, bed-bugs or lice interfered with the acceptability of spraying programmes in endemic communities (Gramiccia & Beales 1988).

The African pilot projects took place in Liberia and in a number of British and French colonies between the mid-1950s and the early 1960s (Harrison 1978). In the pilot areas of Uganda, Liberia and southern Cameroon, malaria transmission was truly interrupted mainly by spraying of residual insecticides, but in the pilot areas of Dahomey (now Benin), Togo, northern Cameroon, northern Nigeria, Senegal, and Upper Volta (now Burkina Faso), malaria transmission was only reduced (Webb 2009b). The projects were however short-lived and after the interventions were stopped, there was much rebound morbidity. Although the results from these not well documented studies varied from an overall good response in tropical forest and highland savannah areas to a rather poor response in the lowland savannah areas, they were followed by the dubious conclusion that the interruption of malaria transmission is in principle feasible in SSA. The African leaders of the soon after independent countries were however not so much convinced about the value of modern control methods, and this was mainly due to cultural resistance to western-directed malaria control strategies (Webb 2009b). This was despite the clear recommendation of the first African Malaria Conference conducted in Kampala, Uganda, in 1950, *"that malaria should be controlled by modern methods as soon as feasible, whatever the original degree of endemicity, and without awaiting the outcome of further experiments"* (WHO 1951).

The success of large pilot projects in Asia together with the important discovery in Greece and later in Sardinia and Cyprus, that an appropriate combination of focal DDT spraying together with stringent epidemiological surveillance was successful in eliminating malaria and that there is thus no need to eliminate the vector populations ("anophelism without malaria"), paved the way to the establishment of the *Global Malaria Eradication Campaign* (Bruce-Chwatt 1988). Moreover, the WHO Expert Committee clearly recommended that DDT spraying should be the main method for malaria control, as the poor state of health service organisation in most of the tropical rural areas prohibited the efficacy of drug-based strategies. However, the document also stated: *"It is not unreasonable to begin planning for world-wide eradication of malaria ... At the present time there are no obvious technical or economic reasons why malaria could not be driven out of the Americas, Europe, Australia and much of Asia, within the next quarter of a century. As regards to tropical Africa the situation is not quite so promising ... one cannot yet foresee the elimination of malaria from Africa in the near future"* (Bruce-Chwatt 1988).

With further recognition of success stories wherever DDT was used on a large scale, and with increasing support from the international community – besides the WHO, the United Nations International Children's Emergency Fund (UNICEF), the United Nations Food and Agriculture Organization (FAO) and the government of the USA strongly supported antimalarial campaigns based on DDT application – global malaria eradication was more and more considered as feasible and criticism was no longer really accepted. The effects of DDT in high-income countries with low malaria transmission intensity were simply projected to underdeveloped tropical countries with very different epidemiology of malaria and their very limited control capacity (Gramiccia & Beales 1988). Finally, there was the strong consideration that only a rapid all-out attack on malaria with DDT could eradicate the disease before this window of opportunity would be closed due to unavoidable insecticide resistance development, and thus the prospect of long-term savings from time-limited eradication as against ongoing control activities would be lost (Gramiccia & Beales 1988). These considerations were reflected in the resolution WHA8.30 of the 8th World Health Assembly in 1955.

## 1.4 The Global Malaria Eradication Campaign (1954-69)

The concept of malaria eradication was thus adopted by the 8th World Health Assembly in 1955 (figure 11), when 46 out of 56 WHO delegates voted in favour of a worldwide programme (Harrison 1978). Two years later, WHO started to technically support and coordinate a *Global Malaria Eradication Campaign* (Najera 1989, Najera 2001). There were, however, some cautionary opinions already heard at the WHO at that time. These concerned the complexity of malaria epidemiology in endemic areas and in particular the unknown feasibility of malaria elimination in SSA, the need for intense cross-border collaboration, and the wish to restrict spraying with residual insecticides to a maximum of six years in a given area (Gramiccia & Beales 1988). At that time however, the impact of insecticide use for agricultural purposes on mosquito resistance development was not considered, which was also caused by the de facto non-cooperation between the

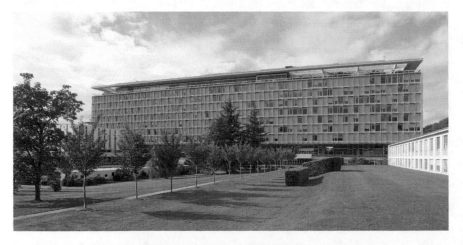

*Figure 11: World Health Organization headquarters in Geneva/Switzerland*
*Source: Wikipedia; www.wikipedia.org/wiki/world health organization, accessed 20.09.2010*

WHO and the FAO and consequent independent policies on insecticides in the health (disease control) and the agricultural (crop protection) sectors (Gramiccia & Beales 1988). Although pilot projects in tropical Asia and Africa did not always showed the expected success, this did not stop the WHO from recommending a malaria eradication approach even in Africa under the expectation that additional control tools would finally stop malaria transmission (Gramiccia & Beales 1988).

The malaria eradication efforts started in all endemic areas at about the same time with strong emphasis on DDT spraying, except in areas with overwhelming technical, financial, social or ecological problems, such as Papua New Guinea, some islands of Indonesia and the whole of tropical Africa, which were unofficially left out (Gramiccia & Beales 1988) (figure 12). It has to be remembered that at the time of the adoption of the eradication concept the African continent was mainly represented by the colonial powers (Harrison 1978). Given the high malaria transmission intensity and the lack of infrastructure in most of SSA, effective implementation of elimination programmes was considered unrealistic, and elimination activities were restricted to countries at the fringe of the continent such as Ethiopia, South Africa and Southern Rhodesia (Zimbabwe), and to a few pilot projects in other areas (Najera 1989, Najera 2001). For endemic areas of countries included into the *Global Malaria Eradication Campaign*, which were hardly accessible and where DDT spraying programmes could not be undertaken, medicated salt programmes with pyrimethaminized or chloroquinized salt provision were developed. The targeted populations in Africa, Asia and Latin America were usually small nomadic or ethnic minority groups of a few hundred to a few thousand people, except in the Amazon Basin of Brazil, where 2.5 million people were included into the medicated salt programme. Interestingly, the places

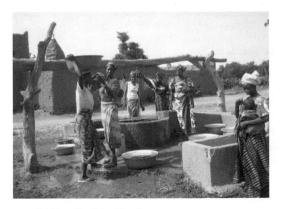

*Figure 12: Village in rural Africa (Burkina Faso)*
*Source: Courtesy Joelle Bals*

33

of later chloroquine resistance development match well with the areas of these medicated salt programmes (Gramiccia & Beales 1988).

The strongly vertical national eradication programmes were typically based on a large-scale application of DDT to interiors of houses and animal shelters, the use of larvicides and environmental measures where appropriate to minimize the populations of infectious *Anopheles* mosquitoes, and – usually towards the end of the attack phase – presumptive treatment of all fever cases and radical treatment (schizontocidal + hypnozoiticidal antimalarials) of confirmed malaria cases. Mass radical treatment was sometimes used to eliminate persistent malaria foci. Programmes were usually carried out over a period of around eight years through a vertical national malaria eradication service, which included a preparatory phase of about 1-2 years duration, an attack phase of 3-4 years duration with a massive application of insecticides, and a consolidation phase with a focus on surveillance which lasted 2-3 years (figure 13). This was then followed by a maintenance phase of variable duration under the responsibility of the national public health services (Onori et al. 1993a).

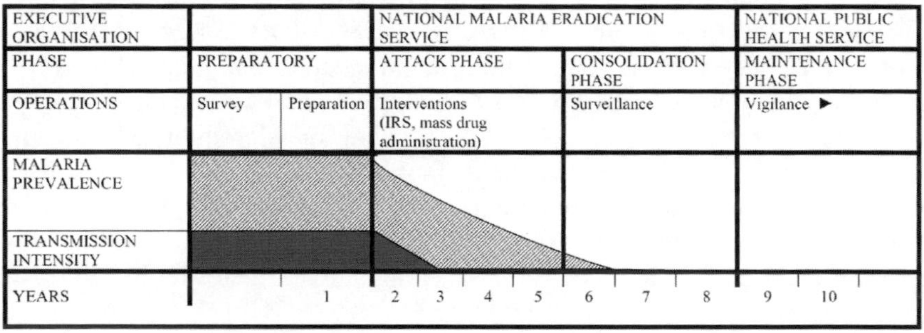

| EXECUTIVE ORGANISATION | | | NATIONAL MALARIA ERADICATION SERVICE | | NATIONAL PUBLIC HEALTH SERVICE |
|---|---|---|---|---|---|
| PHASE | PREPARATORY | | ATTACK PHASE | CONSOLIDATION PHASE | MAINTENANCE PHASE |
| OPERATIONS | Survey | Preparation | Interventions (IRS, mass drug administration) | Surveillance | Vigilance ▶ |
| MALARIA PREVALENCE | | | | | |
| TRANSMISSION INTENSITY | | | | | |
| YEARS | 1 | 2 3 | 4 5 | 6 7 8 | 9 10 |

*Figure 13: Phases of the Global Malaria Eradication Campaign*
*Source: Remade after Bradley (1991)*

At the beginning of the *Global Malaria Eradication Campaign*, countries were proud to participate and money was not a major problem. Unfortunately, this changed considerably when it became obvious that many countries were unable to interrupt malaria transmission which led to costly and sometimes indefinite prolongation of the attack or consolidation phases (Gramiccia & Beales 1988). This was also due to the frequent inability to hand over the programme for the maintenance phase to the weak national public health services. During these early days of the eradication programmes, international and bilateral funding agencies clearly preferred the vertical eradication programmes over horizontal control programmes, which left the highly malaria endemic countries in SSA virtually without international assistance (Gramiccia & Beales 1988). To address this problem, the so-called pre-eradication programmes were created and approved by the 17th World Health Assembly in 1964. These programmes were intended to improve the public health infrastructure and the malaria services in low and middle-income countries, particularly in Africa, including the promotion of research to enable these countries to join the malaria eradication efforts in the future. However, pre-eradication as well as eradication programmes were often not well managed and funds were wasted, but the WHO due to its mandate for coordination and advice could not directly intervene (Gramiccia & Beales 1988). Poor supervision, technical errors and irrational application of insecticides, often accompanied by insecurity, war and civil war, led to persistent malaria transmission in many foci (Harrison 1978). Moreover, some ten years into the Global *Malaria Eradication Campaign,* political support waned and other international public health priorities emerged, namely family planning and smallpox eradication (Gramiccia & Beales 1988). While major efforts to increase family planning services only started during the 1970s, the period of intensification of the *Global Smallpox Eradication Campaign* coincided with the deterioration of the *Global Malaria Eradication Campaign,* and the problem areas of both programmes (South Asia, Indonesia, Brazil, and all of SSA) were largely overlapping (Gramiccia & Beales 1988). In the Brazilian Amazon Region, for example, economic, social, environmental, and political factors produced an epidemiological pattern named „frontier malaria". As the *Global Smallpox Eradication Campaign* received the "highest priority" at the meetings of the World Health Assemblies in 1967, 1968, and 1969, also funds of national malaria eradication programmes were largely diverted towards this new goal (Gramiccia & Beales 1988).

From 1955 until 1974, funds for the *Global Malaria Eradication Campaign* amounted to some 230 million US$ and were provided mainly by WHO and UNICEF (Gramiccia & Beales 1988). The results of the global malaria eradication efforts over these years were excellent for the whole of Europe, the Asian part of the former Soviet Union, several countries in the Middle East, most of North America including the USA, most of the Caribbean, large areas of South America, Australia, Japan, Singapore, Korea, and Taiwan, but less successful – at least in the long-term – in the majority of tropical countries (Onori et al. 1993a, Najera 1989, Najera 2001). In India for example, prior to the eradication programme in 1952, most of the population was at risk from malaria and there were an estimated 75 million malaria cases roughly causing 800,000 deaths per year. About ten years later, more than eighty percent of the population lived in areas where the national malaria eradication programme reached either the maintenance or the consolidation phase and annual malaria morbidity was reduced to less than 100,000 cases with very few deaths (Gramiccia & Beales 1988). However, by 1970 many focal outbreaks were observed and the number of reported malaria cases rapidly increased again, reaching 5.2 million in 1975 (Gramiccia & Beales 1988) (figure 14). In 1997, there were still about 3 million malaria cases with about 1,000 deaths reported from India (Sharma 1999). In Sri Lanka, the number of malaria cases fell from 2.8 million in 1946 to only 17 in 1963, but had reached about half a million cases again by the end of the 1960s with regular epidemics every three to five years (Gramiccia & Beales 1988). Although the low figures initially achieved during the attack phases of the eradication programmes could not be maintained in the poor tropical countries, the resulting endemicity was regularly lower than before the programme had started (Harrison 1978). However, there is quite some uncertainty regarding the validity of malaria estimates in Asia (Hay et al. 2010). While WHO has put annual malaria morbidity at around 10 million cases causing some 15 000 deaths in India, recent evidence points to at least 10 times higher figures (Dhingra et al. 2010).

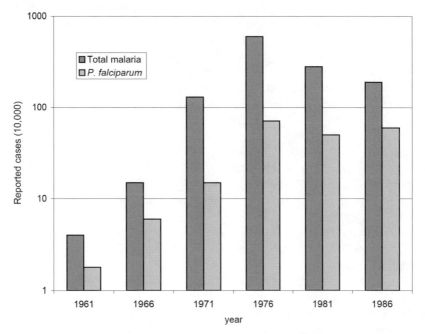

*Figure 14: Malaria resurgence in India after the Global Malaria Eradication Campaign Source: Remade from Bradley (1991)*

The fragility of malaria elimination successes can be illustrated by the case of the island of Mauritius in the Indian Ocean. One of its main malaria vectors, *An. funestus*, was already eradicated with DDT by 1951. During the national elimination campaign, *An. gambiae* was also much reduced, the last indigenous cases of malaria were seen in 1965, and malaria elimination was certified in 1973. However, a devastating cyclone hit Mauritius in 1975, which created many new mosquito-breeding places and led to reintroduction of malaria parasites by foreigners during relief operations. As a result, malaria became endemic again for many years (Gramiccia & Beales 1988).

What were the reasons for the failure of the eradication strategy in most of the underdeveloped countries of the tropics? Amongst the main reasons is the fact that although it was usually possible to significantly reduce malaria transmission by IRS during the attack phases of programmes in those areas, it was much more difficult to establish effective surveillance in the absence of functional health services (Müller 2000). Further important reasons for programme failures included lack of epidemiological expertise and thus local data, lack of transport and other logistical problems particularly in rural areas and during rainy seasons, lack of sufficient community participation, development of insecticide resistance and evasive behaviour of the vector mosquitoes, development of resistance of the parasites to the few available and affordable first-line antimalarial drugs, as well as diverse administrative, socio-economic, financial and political problems (Bruce-Chwatt 1974, Lepes 1974, Ray 1977, Bruce-Chwatt 1984). Moreover, programmes were frequently ineffective in so-called „problem areas", which included remote rural areas with tribal populations, areas of new agricultural exploitation or open mining in jungles, as in the Amazon River basin or the new settlements in the outer islands of Indonesia and other Southeast Asian countries, areas of new agricultural development projects which attracted large labour forces, areas of extensive use of agricultural insecticides followed by rapid resistance development in malaria vectors, border areas with populations engaged in illegal activities, rapidly growing and disorganized periurban slum areas, and areas of socio-political unrest (Najera 1989, Najera 2001).

Only two *Anopheles* species were found to be resistant against DDT in 1946, but this number reached 15 of the relevant malaria vectors in 1968 and 53 by 1991 (Gramiccia & Beales 1988). The extension of resistance from DDT to related compounds (hexachlorocyclohexane, HCH, and dieldrin) questioned the further usefulness of chlorinated hydrocarbons in malaria control, and alternative insecticides proved to be expensive with few tropical countries having been able to afford them. In areas where the principal vector was resistant to DDT, substitution of organophosphorus compounds increased the cost 4-fold, of synthetic pyrethroids 10-fold, and of carbamates 20-fold (Clyde 1987). Moreover, vector resistance against many of the new insecticides also increased rapidly (Onori et al. 1993b).

The large-scale use of proguanil and pyrimethamine monotherapies was accompanied by resistance development of the malaria parasites to these drugs already during the early years of its use (Warrell 1993). This had no major consequences to the *Global Malaria Eradication Campaign* as long as chloroquine remained effective. However, also resistance of *P. falciparum* against chloroquine started to emerge towards the end of the eradication period, and this happened independently in Asia in 1957 and South America in 1959 (Warrell 1993). As one consequence, *P. falciparum* had gradually replaced *P. vivax* as the dominant species in much of Asia (Clyde 1987).

Another problem of the *Global Malaria Eradication Campaign* was the severe neglect of research and training in the field of malaria, due to the confidence in the magic bullet DDT and the hope for rapid eradication (Gramiccia & Beales 1988). It has thus rightly been stated, that the *Global Malaria Eradication Campaign* has finally not been effective in eradicating the disease but the malariologists. Although large numbers of malaria field staff were trained during the time of the global programme activities in specific training centres in collaboration with WHO and USAID for short periods of time (usually one to three months), this did not created much knowledge as these highly standardized trainings only concentrated on basic techniques considered necessary for malaria eradication (Gramiccia & Beales 1988). The result was a generation of desk malariologists who were no longer exposed to laboratory and field experiments, and in fact a separation between malariologists and scientists. Beside the specifically designated *Malaria Eradication Training Centres*, malaria training also took place in national programmes, but again greatly concentrated on eradication and case detection techniques. In addition, large numbers of volunteers were trained nationally for surveillance purposes (Gramiccia & Beales 1988).

Training of sufficient numbers of staff was further complicated by the need for special training and additional staff for subsequent phases of the national malaria eradication programmes. This was often not appropriately budgeted for, and the decreasing malaria burden during the progress of programmes made politicians reluctant to free sufficient funds for the continuation of malaria eradication efforts, in particular in view of the many other pressing health problems. In particular the large number of malaria surveillance agents, who regularly visited their communities during the maintenance phase of respective programmes, was quite expensive and thus hard to sustain (Gramiccia & Beales 1988). As a result, the quality of national programmes deteriorated over time, e.g. due to increasing intervals between insecticide spraying rounds, stopping insecticide spraying prematurely, and neglecting surveillance or even faking results. Thus, the positive spirit of the first years of the *Global Malaria Eradication Campaign* was widely lost (Gramiccia & Beales 1988).

## 1.5 The post-eradication period (1970-2000)

The original enthusiasm for malaria eradication got replaced already by open scepticism by the mid-1960th in view of the multiple technical, managerial and financial problems encountered. It was soon recognised, that the *Global Malaria Eradication Campaign* was only able to eliminate malaria from the European and Australian continent, North America and several small islands, while in the tropics the situation was stagnating or deteriorating (Gramiccia & Beales 1988). At this point in time, the *Malaria Expert Committee of WHO* came up with the following definition for areas of failed programmes: *"Areas with technical problems are those where the planned single or combined attack measures failed to interrupt transmission"* (Gramiccia & Beales 1988). As a consequence, WHO started to invest more into research which led to some limited success, for example in the area of developing new residual insecticides (e.g. organophosphates and carbamates) or new antimalarial drugs (e.g. sulfonamides and sulfones combined with dihydrofolate reductase inhibitors) (Gramiccia & Beales 1988).

In 1968, WHO commissioned an evaluation of the global strategy of malaria eradication through a multidisciplinary team of external experts (Gramiccia & Beales 1988). In 1969, based on the report of this evaluation, the 22nd World Health Assembly abandoned officially the principle of a global time-limited malaria eradication campaign (Trigg & Condrachine 1998). The ultimate goal of malaria eradication was however reaffirmed, but it was emphasised that in regions where elimination did not appear to be feasible, control strategies should be employed (Najera 1989, Najera 2001). Ironically, the terminology "malaria eradication" was from now on widely banned from WHO's official language, similar to the fate of the terminology "malaria control" after the year 1955 (Gramiccia & Beales 1988).

As a consequence of the perceived failure of the eradication approach, the 1970s were characterised by major reductions in internal and external funding for national malaria programmes. This development was further aggravated by the world economic crisis of the 1970s, which resulted in steeply rising costs for drugs and insecticides. As a result of the reductions in antimalarial activities, malaria started a rapid resurgence in many regions of Asia and Latin America (Onori et al. 1993b). In many of the tropical countries which had rolled back malaria dramatically during their attack phases of the *Global Malaria Eradication Campaign*, periodic resurgences were followed by remobilisation of antimalarial activities, after which the situation improved but could not be maintained and was followed by a new resurgence. Such transformations of originally endemic situations into sequences of periodic epidemics were not considered acceptable (Trigg and Condrachine 1998).

In most of the malaria-free countries in the developed world, the risk of a reintroduction of malaria was minimal due to their advanced socio-economic status. However, in countries which experienced a collapse of social services caused by socio-economic degradation and/or socio-political unrest, malaria epidemics were likely to be followed by a reestablishment of malaria endemicity. This has been the case in a number of southern countries (e.g. Azerbaijan, Tajikistan, Georgia, Armenia, Kyrgyzstan) of the former Soviet Union after the end of the cold war in the year 1991, countries where malaria had been successfully eliminated in the early 1960s (Field 1995, WHO 1997). Other reasons for resurgence of malaria were development projects, as it was the case in Turkey following the introduction of large-scale dam building and irrigation (WHO 1997).

The end of the *Global Malaria Eradication Campaign* changed little of the malaria situation in Africa (figure 15). Here and despite somewhat promising results of the pilot projects and the clear recommendation of the first African Malaria Conference in 1950 to use modern control methods in the highly endemic areas of SSA, malaria eradication was never really an explicit goal (Gramiccia & Beales 1988). In subsequent years, the malaria problem appeared to be solved in tropical Africa by increasing the availability of cheap, safe and effective first-line treatment, chloroquine, at least until resistance against this drug started to rise by the end of the 1970s (Kean 1979, Wernsdorfer 1994, Müller et al. 1996). Together with the already huge impact of the AIDS epidemic, the spread of chloroquine resistance was leading to increasing childhood mortality rates in Africa (Marsh 1998, Müller & Garenne 1999, Trapé 2001). As a consequence, some African countries had already changed their drug policy during the 1990s and employed pyrimethamine-sulfadoxine as first-line treatment for uncomplicated malaria, while others were still testing potential alternatives (Bloland et al. 1993, Müller et al. 1996, Müller et al. 2004). In many countries of Southeast Asia and South America the situation was even worse at that time, with multidrug-resistance including resistance to quinine spreading rapidly (White 1992, Hien et al. 1996).

The situation was always different in less endemic and more socio-economically advanced countries of southern Africa. Here, large-scale malaria control programmes based on IRS were already successfully implemented before the *Global Malaria Eradication Campaign* and have continued until today (Mabaso et al 2004). Over the years, these programmes achieved sustainable major reductions in malaria transmission and malaria-attributed morbidity and mortality in countries like South Africa, Swaziland, Botswana, Namibia, Zimbabwe and Mozambique, and this was also associated with an acceleration of economic growth (Mabaso et al 2004). National programmes in these countries used different insecticides, but there was gradual resistance development over time. For instance, in South Africa IRS was conducted with DDT from 1960 until 1996 and with

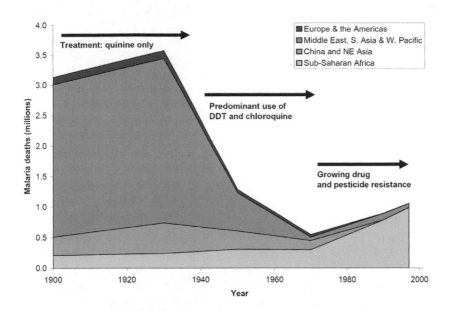

*Figure 15: Global malaria mortality during the 20th century*
*Source: Remade from Carter & Mendis (2002)*

deltamethrin afterwards, but due to resistance development of *An. funestus* it had to be replaced by DDT again in 2000 (Mabaso et al 2004). Although IRS contributed largely to the success of malaria control in southern Africa, improved socioeconomic conditions together with a good public health infrastructure played an important role. However, the fragility of malaria control successes was again demonstrated by the occurrence of increasing numbers of malaria epidemics in this part of Africa since the mid-1980s, which was partly explained by global climatic changes, resistance development of *P. falciparum* against chloroquine and sulphadoxine/pyrimethamine, increasing HIV prevalence, the emergence of pyrethroid resistance, increased migration of malaria carriers, and biological, behavioural and social resistance against IRS with insecticides (Mabaso et al 2004).

The nearly total dependence of malaria control on cheap and effective first-line drugs in SSA was also very much influenced by a few larger and well documented malaria control projects, which followed the pilot projects conducted during the time of the *Global Malaria Eradication Campaign*. One of these projects took place from 1972 to 1976 in Kenya near Kisumu through a collaboration between the WHO and the Government of Kenya (Fontane et al. 1978). This was a multidisciplinary, longitudinal controlled study on the epidemiology and control of malaria in a population of roughly 20,000 in a highly malaria endemic area with perennial transmission on the shores of Lake Victoria. After collection of baseline data, the intervention consisted of eight rounds of IRS with the organophosphorus insecticide fenitrothion over a period of two years. The baseline data confirmed the very high transmission intensity in this rural area, which was virtually without access to modern malaria treatment. IRS rapidly reduced both the malaria vectors and the malaria incidence and prevalence to low levels, but not to zero. This was explained by the partly exophilic behaviour of the *An. gambiae* vectors. The conclusions of the study were that IRS was effective against malaria in SSA, but that it was too expensive for the whole of SSA; elimination may however be achieved with the addition of complimentary interventions such as mass drug administration (MDA) (Fontane et al. 1978).

The best known and documented African project is the Garki Project, which was a proof of principle study, established from 1969 until 1976 in the Garki District of northern Nigeria through a WHO/Government of Nigeria/Kano State collaboration (Molineaux & Gramiccia 1980). This was a well-conducted multidisciplinary, longitudinal study on the epidemiology and control of malaria in a population of roughly 50,000 in the highly malaria endemic Sudan savannah with a seasonal transmission pattern. After collection of baseline data, the intervention consisted IRS with the carbamate insecticide propoxur at intervals of two months before and during the malaria transmission seasons of the years 1972 and 1973 (whole area, 104 villages), of IRS complemented by MDA with sulfalene-pyrimethamine every 10 weeks (subarea 1), and of IRS plus MDA at higher frequency (every two weeks during the rainy season, every 10 weeks during the dry season) plus very limited larviciding with temephos (subarea 2). To avoid harm after the 18 months intervention period, chloroquine treatment was provided to subsequent fever cases. The control area comprised of 5 villages where no interventions took place. Very detailed entomologic, parasitologic, serologic and clinical data were collected at baseline and during followup in representative populations. The results of this study confirmed the high transmission intensity, which showed however large seasonal, annual and local variations, which were partly explained by variations in the exophily of local vectors. IRS reduced the malaria transmission risk by 90 percent, but malaria parasite rates only by 25%; adding MDA reduced parasite rates to low levels, but without being able to interrupt transmission. The conclusions of the study were that – given the high vectorial capacity together with a substantial exophily of the vector mosquitoes – IRS combined with MDA is unable to interrupt malaria transmission and thus not recommended in the Sudan savannah of SSA. The main recommendation for the control of malaria morbidity and mortality was to make chloroquine widely available for treatment of all fever cases (Molineaux & Gramiccia 1980).

In the year 1979, the global status of malaria programmes was evaluated by a WHO expert team. Of 143 countries where malaria had previously been endemic, elimination was completed in 37 countries. In 16 additional countries, the risk of infection was minimised, while in the remaining 90 countries malaria remained a major public health problem (Najera 1989, Najera 2001). In the same year, the 31st World Health Assembly recommended a strategy of malaria control which was in accordance with the principles of the 1978 Conference on Primary Health Care (PHC) in Alma-Ata (WHO/UNICEF 1978). It was expected, that the development of PHC would ensure the necessary structures for the delivery of malaria control measures (Trigg and Condrachine 1998).

In practice, the development of PHC was slow and the integration of antimalarial activities in PHC was not easy (Müller 2000). Existing malaria programs were often reluctant to give up the habits of eradication days and continued with the practice of case detection through microscopical screening of all fever cases, although this no longer carried beneficial consequences. Peripheral health workers were often overloaded with different activities, and they were not well trained and often not adequately supervised for malaria control (Najera 1989, Greenwood 1997, Najera 2001). Malaria eradication had largely eliminated local malaria control capacity, and there was a lack of understanding for the necessity to keep central malaria control units for research and supervision of peripheral health services. Finally, community education and participation was frequently inadequate (Tanner and Vlassoff 1998). For these reasons and aggravated by the continuous increase in resistance of *P. falciparum* against the few available first-line antimalarial drugs, the malaria situation continued to deteriorate during the 1980s and 1990s (Anonymous 1983, WHO 1997, Trigg and Condrachine 1998).

As a consequence of these unfortunate developments, the *Special Programme for Research and Training in Tropical Diseases* (WHO-TDR), a programme co-sponsored by WHO, the United Nations Development Programme (UNDP), and the World Bank, was initiated in 1975 (Ridley & Fletcher 2008). This programme concentrated on the development of new and the improvement of existing tools for the control of tropical diseases including malaria, and the strengthening of institutions to increase the research and training capacities of endemic countries. WHO-TDR has since conducted an invaluable amount of research and training activities, which have bridged the time until new and more powerful international health initiatives have entered the field (Gramiccia & Beales 1988).

Since the early 1990s, malaria has received renewed attention by the international community, and there was and is now a particular consideration of the dramatic malaria situation in Africa (Marsh 1998). The 1992 Ministerial Conference on Malaria in Amsterdam proposed a comprehensive *Global Malaria Control Strategy* which was adopted by the 45th World Health Assembly in 1993, the 1994

United Nations General Assembly and the 1997 Assembly of the Organisation of African Unity (Trigg and Condrachine 1998). The *Global Malaria Control Strategy* called for a disease- rather than a parasite oriented approach, and was based on PHC, decentralisation and multisectoriality (WHO 1993a).

The four technical elements of this strategy were:

- to provide early diagnosis and prompt treatment;
- to plan and implement selective and sustainable preventive measures, including vector control;
- to detect, contain, or prevent epidemics; and
- to strengthen local capacities in basic and applied research to permit and promote the regular assessment of a country's malaria situation, in particular, the ecological, social, and economic determinants of the disease

In malaria-endemic countries of SSA, the actual malaria control priorities have been since on strengthening the capacity for early diagnosis and treatment, management of severe and complicated disease, detection and management of epidemics, and community participation. In endemic countries of Asia, the Americas, and North-Africa, in which organized malaria control activities have been carried out for many decades, priorities have shifted to the strengthening of curative services, promotion of rational drug use, provision of health information, and selective vector control measures (Trigg and Condrachine 1998, Gomes and Salazar 1990, WHO 1993b, Sharma 1999, Gusmao 1999).

# Chapter 2. Epidemiology of malaria in Africa

## 2.1 Introduction

It has been estimated, that of the globally 300-700 million annual clinical malaria cases about 70-80% occur in SSA, and that of the globally 1-3 million annual malaria death about 90% occur in SSA (Müller 2000, Breman et al. 2006) (figure 16). While falciparum malaria dominates in the highly endemic countries of SSA and in a few countries outside Africa such as Haiti and Papua New Guinea, vivax malaria is the main manifestation in Latin America and Asia (Guerra et al. 2010). Globally, the annual incidence of falciparum malaria cases was around 500 million and that of vivax malaria cases around 100 million in the early 21$^{st}$ century, with most of falciparum malaria occurring in SSA and most of vivax malaria occurring outside SSA (Mendis et al. 2001, Snow et al. 2005).

In sharp contrast to most of the malaria endemic areas in Asia and Latin America, malaria is responsible for a large proportion of childhood morbidity and mortality in SSA (Becher et al. 2008, Ndugwa et al. 2008, Black et al. 2010). Up to half of all fever episodes are typically caused by malaria in Africa, but there are large variations in the malaria-attributable fraction depending on endemicity and season (Brinkmann and Brinkmann 1991, Müller 2000, Breman 2006). In the years before RBM, it was estimated that around one quarter of deaths in children aged one to four years in The Gambia were directly caused by malaria (Greenwood et al. 1987). More recently and based on the instrument of verbal autopsy, malaria was estimated to cause about half of all deaths in children under five years of age in rural north-western Burkina Faso (Hammer et al. 2006). Moreover and based on findings from large intervention studies, malaria is also considered a major indirect cause for mortality in young African children (Molineux 1997, Müller 2000). Table 1 shows the most recent estimates of the global malaria morbidity and mortality and the African share of this burden after a few years of a globally intensive roll-out of the available malaria interventions (see also 4.3.4) (WHO 2009b).

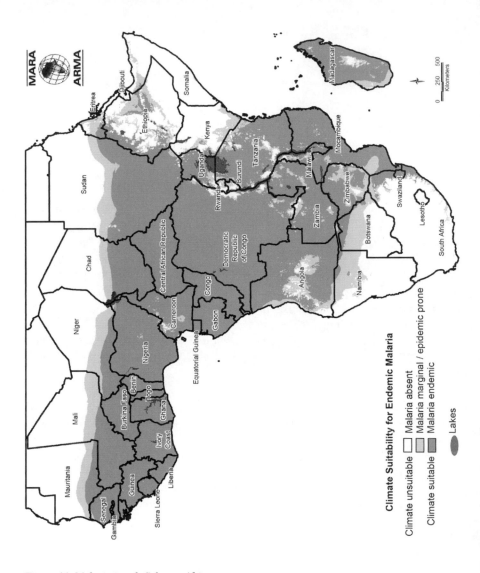

*Figure 16: Malaria in sub-Saharan Africa*
*Source: MARA/ARMA http://www.mara.org.za/ accessed 07.10.10*

|  | Morbidity | falciparum | malaria deaths | children < 5 |
|---|---|---|---|---|
| Global | 243 million | 93% | 863000 | 85% |
| African Region | 208 million | 98% | 767000 | 88% |
|  | 86% |  | 89% |  |

*Table 1: Malaria morbidity and mortality in 2008*

Some 120 different *Plasmodium* parasites exist today, which are responsible for malaria infections in reptiles, birds and mammals (Gilles 1993). Four species of *Plasmodium* parasites cause malaria in humans: *Plasmodium falciparum, P. vivax, P. ovale* and *P. malariae*. Falciparum malaria is caused by *P. falciparum*, which is responsible for most of the global malaria deaths (Greenwood et al. 2005). However, it has become obvious in recent years that also *P. vivax* can lead to severe malaria and significant mortality (Tjitra et al. 2008, Rogerson & Carter 2008, Anstey et al. 2009). More recently, a fifth species has been added – *P. knowlesi* – which occurs sporadically as a zoonosis in countries of South-East Asia (Singh et al. 2004).

Of the more than 400 Anopheles species throughout the world, roughly 70 are malaria vectors, with around 40 of those being of major importance (Müller 2000). The vectorial capacity to transmit malaria is determined by the mean longevity of the local mosquito population, its density in relation to humans, and the frequency of its feeding on humans (anthropophily) as opposed to feeding on animals (zoophily). Further characteristics of vector importance are the habit of obtaining the blood meal outside (exophagy) or inside (endophagy) of houses, as well as preference for resting inside (endophily) or outside (exophily) houses (Müller 2000). *Anopheles* breeding places vary from fresh to brackish water, from standing water to open streams, from water in open sun to water in deep shade, and from large open marshes to tiny pools of water (Clyde 1987, Service 1993, Onori et al. 1993b). In SSA, the *An. gambiae* complex and *An. funestus* are the most important malaria vectors which carry an extraordinary high vectorial capacity.

Regions can roughly be classified into regions of endemic or stable and regions of epidemic or unstable malaria (Müller 2000). The classical epidemiological malaria prototypes are (1) African savannah, (2) desert fringe and highland fringe,

(3) malaria associated with traditional agriculture in plains and river valleys outside Africa, (4) forest-related malaria, (5) malaria associated with extensive agricultural development, (6) urban malaria, (7) coastland and marshland malaria and (8) malaria in war zones and areas with socio-political disturbances (Gilles 1993). Vector control measures are usually considered more difficult against African savannah malaria due to vector density as well as against forest-related malaria due to highly exophilic vectors (Müller 2000). With rapidly increasing urbanisation, urban malaria is becoming more important in all of SSA (Breman et al. 2006).

The endemicity of malaria is defined traditionally in terms of the spleen or parasite rates in children aged between 2 and 9 years (White 2009).

- Hypoendemic: spleen rate or parasite rate 0-9%
- Mesoendemic: spleen rate or parasite rate 10-49%
- Hyperendemic: spleen rate or parasite rate 50-75% and adult spleen rate also high
- Holoendemic: spleen rate or parasite rate above 75% and adult spleen rate low. Parasite rates in the first year of life are high.

Malaria epidemics are typically caused by an increase in the proportion of non-immune individuals in the population of an endemic region, or by a more intense contact of the population with the vector mosquitoes. Climatic changes play an important role in the development of malaria epidemics. In SSA, epidemics occur primarily at the fringes of deserts and highlands, but also in areas of new development projects, and areas of war and civil war with massive population movements (Müller 2000).

## 2.2 Parasite populations

### 2.2.1 *Plasmodium falciparum*

During bites of an infected mosquito, an inoculation of a relatively small number of sporozoites (usually 8-15) takes place, which rapidly enter the liver (White 2009). The pre-erythrocytic phase of development in the liver is completed in around a week (5-7 days). The following erythrocytic schizogony in *P. falciparum* usually takes 48 hours leading to a typical tertian type pattern of symptom occurrence (Gilles 1993). However, due to the reality of frequent infections with more than one brood of parasites and subsequent lack of synchronisation, the periodicity of symptoms is often irregular in falciparum malaria. The gametocytes of *P. falciparum* usually occur in the peripheral blood some ten days after the beginning of the invasion of erythrocytes has started (Gilles 1993). The duration of the sexual cycle in the mosquito is strongly temperature-dependant and varies between 22 days at 20°C and 9 days at 28°C (Gilles 1993). *P. falciparum* is confined to tropical and subtropical areas due to the requirement of temperatures above 20°C (figure 17).

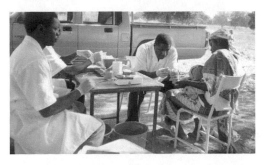

*Figure 17: Malaria survey conducted in the research zone of the Centre de Recherche en Santé de Nouna in rural north-western Burkina Faso*

*P. falciparum* is the far most prevalent malaria parasite in SSA (Snow et al. 1999). In the non-immune human host, the parasite multiplies rapidly and affects all stages of the erythrocytes. Without early effective treatment, this usually leads to high parasite densities of up to several 100.000 parasites per µl blood. The older parasites usually disappear from the peripheral blood and sequester in the capillaries of internal organs where they further develop under relative protection from the immune system (Gilles 1993). These specificities are the main reasons for the severe clinical manifestations of falciparum malaria (White 2009).

It has been estimated that some 2.37 billion people were at some risk for falciparum malaria in 2007, with 0.61 billion living in the African Region (Guerra et al. 2007) (figure 18). The African continent can epidemiologically be stratified into northern, eastern, western, central and southern Africa, but also into areas of stable or unstable malaria transmission (Snow et al. 1999). While malaria does virtually no longer exist in northern Africa it is highly endemic in most of SSA, with the exception of deserts and highland areas, particularly in eastern Africa, and the less endemic southern part of the continent. In the high transmission settings of African savannah areas, typically some 95 percent or more of all malaria infections are caused by *Plasmodium falciparum* (Müller et al. 2001).

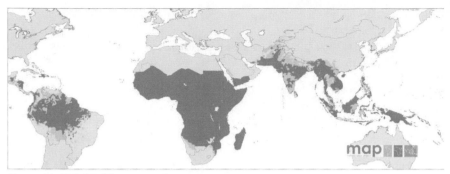

*Figure 18: Global P. falciparum risk*
*(Dark grey areas = stable transmission; middle grey areas = unstable transmission; light grey areas = no transmission)*
*Source: Guerra et al. (2008)*

## 2.2.2 *Plasmodium vivax*

The sporozoites of this parasite differentiate either into primary tissue schizonts or into hypnozoites after liver invasion. The primary tissue schizonts also complete the pre-erythrocytic phase of development in the liver in around a week (6-8 days). The duration of the following erythrocytic schizogony in *P. vivax* is 48 hours, leading to a typical tertian type pattern of symptom occurrence (Gilles 1993). The dormant hypnozoite form of the parasite is responsible for relapse of infection, which may occur already after a few weeks or only after several months in tropical and northern strains of *P. vivax* respectively. The merozoites of *P. vivax* predominantly infect the young erythrocytes and parasite densities are usually lower as compared to *P. falciparum*. The gametocytes of *P. vivax* usually occur in the peripheral blood within three days after red blood cell invasion (Gilles 1993). The duration of the sexual cycle in the mosquito takes 16 days at 20°C and 8-10 days at 28°C (Gilles 1993).

It has been estimated that some 2.85 billion people were at some risk for vivax malaria in 2009, but only 3.5% of those were living in the Africa Region (Guerra et al. 2010) (figure 19). *P. vivax* is rare in Africa, particularly in western Africa, due to the high prevalence of the Duffy negative trait, an inherited red cell phenotype that lacks the receptor for invasion of the human erythrocyte by the *P. vivax* parasite (Mendis et al. 2001). *P. vivax* has been estimated to represent less than one percent of the malaria infections in SSA, but around 20 percent of malaria cases are caused by this parasite in eastern and southern Africa, and in Madagascar (Mendis et al. 2001, Guerra et al. 2010).

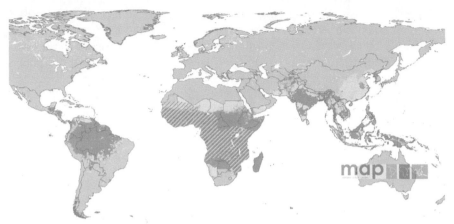

*Figure 19: Global P. vivax risk*
*(Dark areas = stable transmission; light grey areas = unstable transmission; middle grey areas =*
*no transmission; hatched areas = Duffy negativity prevalence >90%)*
*Source: Guerra et al. (2010)*

### 2.2.3 *Plasmodium ovale*

This parasite is the cause of a tertian type of malaria fever similar to that of vivax malaria, but often with prolonged latency, less frequent relapses and a milder clinical presentation (Gilles 1993). *P. ovale* mainly occurs in SSA and in particular in western Africa, but has also been reported sporadically from Asia. In a savannah area of north-western Burkina Faso, 10% of malaria infections in young children had detectable *P. ovale* parasites in the peripheral blood with the great majority being mixed infections with *P. falciparum* (Müller et al. 2001).

### 2.2.4 *Plasmodium malariae*

This parasite causes the quartan malaria, which is characterised by fever episodes every fourth day caused by erythrocytic schizogony after 72 hours (Gilles 1993). The parasite density is usually low and the clinical development not severe, but an untreated infection can persist for a very long time and probably for a lifetime. This is despite the fact that *P. malariae* does not develop hypnozoites and is thus unable to present with true relapses. Quartan malaria is found in SSA but also in various malaria endemic countries outside Africa (Gilles 1993). In rural north-western Burkina Faso, 6% of malaria infections in young children had detectable

51

*P. malariae* parasites in the peripheral blood with the great majority being mixed infections with *P. falciparum* (Müller et al. 2001).

*P. malariae* occurs naturally in chimpanzees which may form a natural reservoir for this type of malaria. Thus, malaria caused by *P. malariae* is by definition a zoonosis. That malaria in humans is to a certain degree a zoonosis is furthermore supported by the recent detection of another *Plasmodium* species *(P. knowlesi)* – which usually affects primates – being able to cause disease and death in humans (Singh et al. 2004, Galinski & Barnwell 2009).

## 2.3 Vector populations

### 2.3.1 *Anopheles gambiae*

Within a species group of some *Anopheles* mosquitoes there are forms with distinct biological characteristics (figure 20). This is of practical importance as the different members of such *species complexes* differ markedly in their feeding, resting and other types of behaviour, which is relevant for malaria control considerations (Burkot & Graves 2000). *Anopheles gambiae* clearly is the most important malaria vector in SSA and is a complex of a number of sibling species (Service 1993). The *Anopheles gambiae* complex is the major vector system in Africa and exists only in frost-free regions, or where the minimum temperature in winter remains above 5°C (Snow *et al.* 1999). Of the relevant vectors in this complex, three *(An. gambiae sensu stricto, An. arabiensis, An. bwambae)* are adapted to fresh-water and two *(An. melas, An. merus)* to salt-water breeding sites. *An. gambiae s.s.* predominates in humid areas, is highly anthropophilic and endophilic, and is the far most important malaria vector. *An. arabiensis* prefers more the not so humid savannah areas, is often more zoophilic and exophilic, but is also considered as an important malaria vector. All malaria vectors bite at night, with *An. gambiae s.s.* being most active between 2.00 and 4.00 in the morning. *An. gambiae s.s.* and *An. arabiensis* breed in various water bodies but clearly avoid shadow. These are frequently small and temporary water collections such as pools, puddles, borrow pits, hoof prints, and all kind of man-made containers, but also permanent and larger water bodies such as ponds, swamps and rice fields (Service 1993, Fillinger et al. 2009a). As a consequence, there occur multiple breeding places during the rainy season which are impossible to be controlled by environmental measures or larviciding at least in the rural areas of SSA. *An. bwambae* only exists very focally in the Rift Valley of East Africa, where it breads in geothermal water (Service 1993). Of the two salt-water species,

*An. melas* is found in West Africa and *An. merus* in east Africa. They are more exophagic and zoophilic and thus poorer vectors compared to *An. gambiae s.s.* (Service 1993). In most of SSA, the *An. gambiae* complex is found as a mixed population without interbreeding.

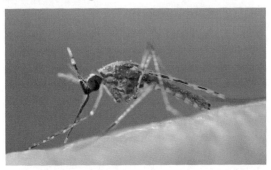

*Figure 20: Anopheles stephensi during blood meal*
*Source: Courtesy Mirko Merkel*

In The Gambia, an entomological survey showed that 98% of the mosquitoes collected with "spray catches" inside houses were members of the *An. gambiae* complex (Lindsay et al. 1993). In the Dielmo site of Senegal, *An. gambiae* s.s. represented 62% of the 11.685 anopheles collected in 1990-1992 and was abundant mainly in the wet season (Trape *et al.* 1994). This vector was responsible for the peak of transmission intensity during the rainy season, with a maximum of 90.5 bites per person per night recorded in September. In the dry season, the density of this vector was generally low (0.9 bites per person per night). The rate of *An. gambiae s.s.* attributed endophagy in this study area was 53% (Trape *et al.* 1994).

In six representative villages of rural north-western Burkina Faso, out of 7.594 mosquitoes caught with "spray catches" inside houses over a period of one year in 2000/2001, 6.598 (87%) were malaria vectors; of the vector mosquitoes, 5.811 (88%) belonged to the *An. gambiae* complex (Traoré 2003). Subspecies analysis in a random subsample demonstrated An. *gambiae* s.s. being the predominant vector (46/50=92%), beside *An. arabiensis* (4/50=8%).

### 2.3.2 *Anopheles funestus*

*An. funestus,* the other major vector in the afrotropical zone, prefers shaded habitats and breeds in permanent waters, especially with vegetation, such as marshes, grassy edges of streams, rivers and ditches, and rice fields with mature plants providing shade. Due to the nature of its breeding places, *An. funestus* often becomes

53

the main malaria vector during the dry season in many areas of SSA, whereas *An. gambiae* is of major importance during the rainy season. The optimum water temperature for the larvae of *An. funestus* is 18-20°C and they do not like higher water temperatures. It bites humans predominantly but also domestic animals, and is exophagic and endophagic (Service 1993).

In the study conducted over a one year period in rural north-western Burkina Faso, out of the 6.598 *Anopheles* mosquitoes, 538 (8%) were *An. funestus* (Traoré 2003).

### 2.3.3 Vectorial capacity

The vectorial capacity describes the number of new malaria infections disseminated per day by each vector mosquito that has fed on an infected person. It is determined by (1) the human biting rate (bites per person per night), (2) the human blood index (proportion of blood meals taken from humans), (3) the vector competence of the mosquito for the parasite, (4) the daily survival rate of the vector, and (5) the extrinsic incubation period for the malaria parasite in the vector (Burkot & Graves 2000).

Methods used to estimate the human biting rate include "spray catches", "landing rates" and "exit" and "bed net traps". These methods do partly over- or underestimate the true biting rates (Bukot & Graves 2000). The human blood index is determined by immunologic or molecular-based methods which identify the source of the blood meal. Mosquito survival can be estimated as the proportion of adult female mosquitoes surviving per time period (e.g. per day or feeding cycle) and is difficult to measure. The extrinsic incubation period for the malaria parasite in the vector varies from 10-30 days, depending on temperature and parasite species. However, it has been demonstrated in high transmission settings that the length of the feeding cycle, and therefore the number of feeding cycles per extrinsic incubation period, varies with season and location (Lindsay et al. 1991).

Studies have identified components of the vectorial capacity with better correlation to parasite measurements in humans than overall estimates of vectorial capacity, such as the entomological inoculation rate (EIR) (Burkot & Graves 2000). The EIR is a commonly used but poorly standardised measure of malaria transmission intensity (Kelly-Hope & McKenzie 2008). It measures the number of infective bites per person per time unit (number of vector bites multiplied with the fraction of vector mosquitoes that are infectious). The infectiousness is determined by measuring the sporozoite rate of the mosquitoes, usually with immunological methods.

Among the factors affecting the transmission of malaria parasites to vector mosquitoes are the proportion of persons who have gametocytes in their blood, the density of the gametocytaemia, the gametocyte infectivity, and the susceptibility of the specific mosquito to become infected (Burkot & Graves 2000). Some antimalarials such as primaquine, artemisinin derivates and methylene blue have a high capacity to suppress gametocyte prevalence and density and may thus contribute to significant reductions of malaria transmission (Baird 2008, International Artemisinin Study Group 2009, Coulibaly et al. 2009).

In the large study conducted in the Nouna area of north-western Burkina Faso, out of 5.247 *P. falciparum* sporozoite ELISA results, 385 (7.3%) were positive (Traoré 2003). Sporozoite rates varied largely by village and season, with highest rates (around 10%) observed towards the end of the rainy season between September and November. Estimates in EIR rates varied in the six villages surveyed between 100 and 1000 per year (Traoré 2003). In the central region of Burkina Faso, a study on the EIR variations between villages showed variations from 82 to 442 infective bites per person per year in 1984 (Hay *et al.* 2000). A recent review on annual EIRs attributed to *P. falciparum* in 23 countries of Africa calculated an average EIR of 112 (ranging from 0.6 in Sudan to 814 in Equatorial Guinea), thus demonstrating the overall high malaria transmission intensity in most of SSA (Kelly-Hope & McKenzie 2008).

## 2.4 Human populations

### 2.4.1 Clinical manifestations

Malaria is an acute illness with more or less periodic febrile paroxysms. In its mild form, malaria presents as a febrile illness associated with other non specific signs and symptoms (Warrell 1993). No clinical syndrome is entirely specific for malaria, and particularly in children symptoms often mimic other common diseases (Müller et al. 1996). The severity and course of an acute attack of malaria depends on many factors, such as (1) the species and the strain of the infecting parasite, (2) the age and the specific immunity of the affected individual, (3) the general health status and the genetic constitution of the patient, (4) the type of previous chemoprophylactic or chemotherapeutic regimens, and (5) how rapid effective treatment is provided.

The incubation period (interval between infection and first clinical signs) and the pre-patent period (interval between infection and the first detection of malaria parasites in the blood) under natural transmission conditions vary between the different malaria species (Warrell 1993, Gilles 1993, White 2009) (table 2). The incubation period is prolonged in subjects with semi-immunity and those who have taken not fully effective chemoprophylaxis or treatment. After unspecific prodromal symptoms 2-3 days before a malaria attack, the disease typically starts with the *cold stage* with a sudden feeling of cold and extensive shivering (Warrell 1993). The temperature is rising quickly, the pulse is rapid, the skin is cold, dry and pale, and the patient may start vomiting or febrile convulsions may develop in case of young children. This cold stage lasts for 15-60 minutes before the *hot stage* begins, which is characterised by feeling hot, headache, palpitations, tachypnoea, prostration and vomiting. This *hot stage* lasts from 2-6 hours and is accompanied by profuse sweating. The fever declines over the following few hours, the symptoms diminish and the patient falls asleep. The duration of such an attack is usually 8-12 hours. The interval between the malaria attacks depends on the length of the asexual erythrocytic cycle, with paroxysms every 48 hours in *P. falciparum, P. vivax* and *P. ovale* (tertian fever) and every 72 hours in *P. malariae* (quartan fever). However, the classical febrile malarial paroxysm with clear periodicity is rarely seen in falciparum malaria, where the illness often starts with headache, dizziness, joint pain, malaise, vomiting and diarrhoea and where daily fever spikes are more usual (Warrell 1993).

*Relapses* in *P. vivax* and *P. ovale* are often triggered by cold, fatigue, trauma, pregnancy or other infections. They result from reactivation of the hypnozoites in the liver. *Recrudescences* result from exacerbations of persistent undetectable parasitaemia in the absence of an exo-erythrocytic cycle (Warrell 1993).

|  | *P. falciparum* | *P. malariae* | *P. vivax* | *P. ovale* |
|---|---|---|---|---|
| Incubation period (days) | 9-14 | 18-40 | 12-17 | 10-14 |
| Fever periodicity (hours) | 24, 36, 48 | 72 | 48 | 48 |
| Relapses | – | – | + | + |
| Recrudescences | + | + | + | + |

*Table 2: Characteristics of the human malaria species*

In the highly endemic areas of SSA and until very recently, malaria was usually diagnosed clinically and only rarely confirmed by the diagnosis of the parasite in the peripheral blood. However, in these areas there are many more asymptomatic carriers of the parasite than symptomatic cases. Hence even parasitological diagnosis does not necessarily indicate that malaria is the cause of the disease (Greenwood *et al.* 1987). A quantitative framework for the analysis has been proposed estimating probabilities that fever episodes are indeed of malaria aetiology as a function of parasite density (Smith *et al.* 1994, Smith et al. 1995). However, in practice more pragmatic parasite thresholds such as 2000 or 5000 parasites per µl are used in malaria studies.

Severe life threatening malaria (e. g. cerebral malaria, respiratory distress, severe anaemia, pulmonary oedema, renal failure) and death is almost exclusively attributed to *P. falciparum* malaria, with young children and pregnant women being the main risk groups in endemic areas (Greenwood et al. 2005) (figure 21). Severe anaemia is defined as haemoglobin < 5 g/dl or haematocrit < 15% (WHO 2000). Cerebral malaria, respiratory distress and severe anaemia are the principle reasons for hospital admission of young children with malaria in endemic areas, while pulmonary oedema and renal failure are manifestations of severe disease

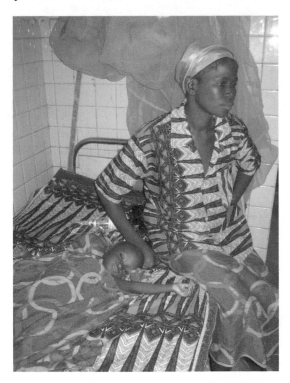

*Figure 21: Child with severe malaria anaemia in Nouna Hospital in Burkina Faso*
*Source: Olaf Müller*

predominantly seen in adults (White 2009). In young children and other non-immune populations, the disease is progressing very rapidly to life-threatening malaria if not treated immediately and with effective drugs. However, clinical diagnosis of malaria in endemic areas is rather complicated as the symptoms of acute respiratory infections and malaria do largely overlap in young children (Marsh et al. 1995). Moreover, coinfection with bacteria is frequently observed during malaria attacks of children and has been shown to be a strong risk factor for mortality (English et al. 1996, Berkley et al. 1999, Berkley 2005). The frequency and pattern of distribution of severe forms of *P. falciparum* malaria vary depending on the level of transmission intensity (Greenwood et al. 2005). Epidemiological studies have shown that under conditions of intense, perennial and stable transmission, severe anaemia is the dominating manifestation of severe malaria, while under conditions of less intense, more seasonal and unstable or epidemic transmission, cerebral malaria becomes the main manifestation of severe malaria in children (Snow *et al.* 1999) (figure 22). The mean age of children with these two syndromes is quite different; severe anaemia affects predominantly infants and children below three years of age while the mean age of children

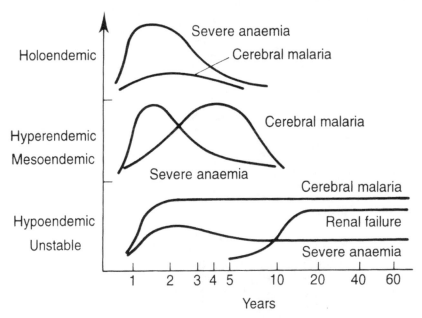

*Figure 22: Relation between malaria endemicity, age and severe malaria*
*Source: White (2009)*

with cerebral malaria is higher (about four years) (Brewster and Greenwood 1993, Snow and Marsh, 1995). In a comparative study of the presentation of severe malaria in urban and rural areas of Burkina Faso characterised by different levels of transmission, Modiano and others found that the prevalence of cerebral malaria was higher in the urban sample (53,6% versus 28,9%) while that of severe anaemia was higher in the rural patients (47,4% versus 14,8%). The urban area was characterised by relatively low transmission (1 to 10 infective bites per person per year), while the EIR in rural zones was 50 to 200 infective bites per person per year (Modiano et al. 1998). It has been projected, that with decreasing transmission intensity the mean age of cerebral malaria will increase but severe anaemia and respiratory manifestations will remain dominant in children under the age of five years (Roca-Feltrer et al. 2010). Anaemia may develop rapidly during the course of the malaria illness, or may be present in a child with cerebral malaria or any other complication of *P. falciparum* infection. Severe anaemia is often multifactorial (WHO 2000, Calis et al. 2008). In a large cohort study in rural north-western Burkina Faso, malnutrition but not malaria was the main cause of anaemia in young children during the rainy season (Müller et al. 2003).

Congenital and neonatal malaria is defined as parasitaemia in the neonate within seven days or later if there is no possibility of post-partum infection by mosquito bite or blood transfusion. It is not uncommon in endemic areas but is rare under conditions of high transmission intensity. It occurs in newborns of up to 0.3% of immune mothers and up to 7.4% of non-immune mothers (MacGregor 1984). Infants of non-immune mothers are more likely to experience symptomatic disease, which typically manifests at 4-6 weeks of life with fever, vomiting, anaemia, hepatosplenomegaly, jaundice and mild diarrhoea (Molyneux 1989). Nevertheless, in a study in a highly endemic area of Tanzania, a proportion of 5,3% congenital malaria was found, and the youngest person who had an attack in an endemic area of Senegal was a two-month-old baby with a parasitaemia of 102.000/ml (Kitua *et al.* 1996, Trape *et al.* 1994).

Until today, the great majority of malaria deaths are in children up to five years old who live in areas of intense transmission of *P. falciparum*, especially in SSA (WHO 1997). In many parts of rural Africa, measuring malaria mortality from statistical records is difficult since 90% of deaths occur at home and are not registered in any formal way (Greenwood, 1999). The only available sources of information on levels of malaria mortality in endemic areas are (Snow and Marsh, 1995):

(1) Conclusions drawn from intensive malaria control studies
(2) Statistical records from existing health services
(3) Data from circumscribed populations under continuous demographic surveillance

Based on such available data, malaria-specific mortality has been estimated in the recent past to have been between 6 and 11 per 1000 children under five years per annum in malaria endemic areas of SSA (Snow & Marsh 1995). In the existing *Demographic Surveillance System* (DSS) areas, overall mortality rates can be measured by active demographic surveillance, while estimation of cause-specific mortality rates depends upon use of post-mortem questionnaire (Brewster and Greenwood 1993, Greenwood 1999). A DSS (which is now called *Health and Demographic Surveillance System*, HDSS), which operates in a circumscribed geographical area, starts with an initial census of the population followed by subsequent regular rounds of data collection on births, deaths, and migrations (INDEPTH Network, 2002). All reported deaths are examined through verbal autopsy interviews conducted after the HDSS rounds. The post-mortem diagnosis can often be achieved by use of an algorithm based on the presence of certain symptoms and signs, the age of the decedent, and the timing of the onset and duration of symptoms/signs during the terminal illness (Snow *et al.*1992). The identification of deaths in early infancy is particularly challenging; pregnancy registration during HDSS rounds and surveillance using community informants are useful methods to identify child deaths before six months of age.

Each year between 75.000 and 200.000 infant deaths are attributed to malaria infection in pregnancy globally, and between 200.000 and 500.000 (of approximately 25 million pregnant women at risk) develop severe anaemia as a result of malaria in SSA (Steketee et al. 2001, Gies 2009). Pregnant women as compared to non-pregnant women are at an increased risk for malaria in endemic areas, and the severity of the clinical manifestations in the women and her foetus depends on the level of pre-pregnancy immunity (Menendez 1995, White 1996). While in areas of low malaria endemicity all pregnant women are equally susceptible to the consequences of malaria infection, in areas of high endemicity women appear to be most susceptible during their first pregnancy, but this susceptibility appears to wane with subsequent pregnancies (Garner and Brabin 1994, Steketee et al. 1996, Bouvier et al. 1997a). Although most infections are asymptomatic in malaria endemic regions, pregnancies in women are associated with *P. falciparum* parasitaemia, with maternal morbidity including severe anaemia, with abortion and stillbirth, and with high rates of placental malaria and consequently low birth weight in newborns caused by intrauterine growth retardation (Garner and Brabin 1994, Steketee et al. 1996, Bouvier et al. 1997a, Bouvier et al. 1997b, Shulman et al. 2001). Malaria during pregnancy thus significantly contributes to maternal and infant mortality in endemic regions (Menendez 1995, McDermott et al. 1996, Slutsker et al. 1996, Bloland et al. 1996).

## 2.4.2 Immunity development

The immune response to malaria is very complex and still incompletely understood. Also the relative contributions of humoral and cellular immunity mechanisms are not yet defined clearly (White 2009). However, it is obvious from experimental studies in humans in the last century that strain-specific immunity can rapidly be achieved but does not protect against different malaria strains. Moreover, antigenic variation of the parasite proteins expressed on the red cell surface protects the parasites from complete clearance. Effective semi-immunity, which develops from antitoxic to antiparasitic immunity, is reached after exposure to all local strains of the dominating malaria species has taken place (White 2009). This is usually the case after the first few years of childhood in hyper/holoendemic areas and takes longer under conditions of less intense transmission intensity (Greenwood et al. 2005).

In highly malaria endemic areas, young infants as compared to older children are relatively protected against all forms of malaria, an effect mainly achieved through foetal haemoglobin and passively transferred maternal antibodies (Snow *et al.* 1998). This protection usually lasts for 4-6 months after which the infants become increasingly susceptible to malaria disease and deaths (Traoré 2003). The highest incidence of severe malaria and associated mortality thus occurs in the second half of infancy under conditions of high malaria transmission intensity (Hammer et al. 2006).

The relation between malaria immunity development, transmission intensity, and morbidity and mortality is rather complicated. Existing data on this topic have been discussed very controversially because of their important consequences for the current roll out of existing malaria control tools in the whole of SSA (Müller 2000).

Data on this topic have been published from Senegal, where the number of malaria attacks were compared between Dakar (1 infective bite per person per year), Dip (20 infective bites per person per year) and Dielmo (200 infective bites per person per year). Despite such major differences in transmission intensity, the cumulative number of malaria attacks by the age of 60 years was pretty similar – 30, 62 and 43 respectively. These fluctuations show that major variations in malaria transmission intensity have been associated only with minor variations in malaria morbidity (Trape & Rogier 1996). This deduction is supported by findings from Tanzania where each 10-fold increase in the EIR corresponded to only a 1.6-fold increase of incidence of clinical malaria (Smith *et al.* 1998). Quantifying the relationship between transmission levels and the incidence of clinical attacks, Trape and Rogier found that for low levels of transmission, i.e. between 0.001 and 0.1 infective bites per person per year, the incidence of malaria attacks is probably directly proportional to the level of transmission. For levels of transmission of 1, 10, 100 and 1000 infective bites per person per year, the data suggest that the number of malaria attacks varies at maximum by a factor of two to three according to the level of transmission (Trape & Rogier 1996).

A number of studies have been focused on the relationship between the intensity of malaria transmission and severe disease and mortality. A study in East Africa which compared the pattern of malaria disease in Kilifi (0-60 infective bites per person per year) and Ifakara (10-3000 infective bites per person per year) revealed that children with malaria in Ifakara were younger and that there were three times more cases of severe anaemia, while cases of cerebral malaria were four times more frequent in Kilifi. Despite these major differences the overall rate of severe disease among children under five years were not very different (Snow et al. 1995). In accordance with these findings, studies from the Republic of Congo showed very little variation in malaria mortality despite extreme differences (0.3-100 infective bites per person per year) in malaria transmission intensity (Trape & Rogier 1996). However, malaria mortality in the Republic of Congo was lower as compared to similar epidemiological areas, and this was attributed to the ready available malaria drugs in this urban setting (Carme 1996). The most provocative findings were published by Snow and colleagues in the year 1997 (see also 3.2.6). In this study rates of severe malaria were compared in two countries of SSA, and the risk of severe disease was lowest in the areas with the highest EIR (Snow et al. 1997). However, the results of Snow et al were subsequently challenged by the documentation of a positive association between the incidence of clinical malaria and EIR even under conditions of very high transmission intensity in young children of rural Tanzania (Kitua 1996).

### 2.4.3 Health seeking behaviour

Treatment-seeking behaviour can be defined as *"any activity undertaken by individuals who perceive themselves to have a health problem or to be ill for the purpose of finding an appropriate remedy"* (Ward et al. 1997). The success of malaria treatment strategies is closely linked to the behaviour of patients and particularly parents of young children. Treatment-seeking behaviour usually depends on the local epidemiology of malaria, access to health care providers, costs of services, attitudes towards providers, perceived severity of disease, age, sex, educational level, socio-economic status, and cultural beliefs about the cause and cure of illness (Deming et al. 1989, Greenwood 1989, Reuben 1993, McCombie 1994, Tanner & Vlassoff 1998, Molyneux et al. 1999, Baume et al. 2000). Although it has been suggested that fever is more likely than other symptoms to prompt caregivers to seek treatment in formal health services, self-medication with drugs purchased from pharmacies and drug sellers is consistently the most common response when people first experience symptoms that could be malaria (Dabis et al. 1989, McCombie 1994). Several studies showed that home treatment and self-medication is common for uncomplicated malaria throughout Africa (Holtz et al. 2003, Sirima et al. 2003, Leonard 2005, Ruebush et al. 1995, Deressa et al. 2003). Such pattern are supported by the results of a large cohort study on treatment seeking behaviour for fever episodes in children living in a malaria holoendemic rural area of Burkina Faso, where the great majority of children were not treated in formal health services (Müller et al. 2003) (table 3). Underdosing of antimalarials received through public or private sector providers is virtually universal, and costs, side-effects and resistance development of drugs used are of increasing concern (McCombie 1994, Ruebush et al. 1995, Tanner & Vlassoff 1998, Baume et al. 2000, Nshakira et al. 2002).

| Treatment category | Household/village (%) | Health Centre/hospital (%) |
|---|---|---|
| Chloroquine | 89 | 11 |
| Antipyretics | 87 | 13 |
| Traditional remedies | 100 | 0 |
| Oral rehydration solution | 46 | 54 |
| Tetracycline | 100 | 0 |
| Qinine | 51 | 49 |
| Ampicillin/amoxycillin | 10 | 90 |
| Cotrimoxazole | 17 | 83 |
| Pyrimethamine-sulfadoxine | 0 | 100 |

*Table 3: Fever treatment in children of rural Burkina Faso*

Medical pluralism also plays an important role with regard to treatment seeking behaviour (Tipke 2010). The understanding and perception of a disease can differ very much from one culture to another. Different names exist throughout different populations to what is called, in a biomedical sense, "malaria". These local names often refer to the main symptom of the disease (Agyepong 1992, Aikins *et al* 1993). In The Gambia, the principal name *Fula kajeho* means « Fula hot body » (Aikins *et al.* 1993). In Ghana, malaria is locally called *Asra or Atridi* and several signs and symptoms are used to recognise this disease entity, e.g. headache, yellowish urine, 'hot body' (locally called *hedora*) (Ahorlu *et al.* 1997). In

Burkina Faso, the term malaria refers to the following categories (Beiersmann et al. 2007):

- *Soumaya:* this represents uncomplicated malaria (fever, vomiting, fatigue, shivering)
- *Dusukun yelema:* this represents complicated malaria (acidosis)
- *Kono:* this represents complicated malaria (cerebral malaria)
- *Djoliban*: this represents complicated malaria (severe anaemia)

These different perceptions have consequences for treatment seeking behaviour. In many African societies illnesses that are believed to be caused by natural conditions (i.e. God-given) are treated within the formal health system, while diseases believed to be caused by unnatural causes (i.e. witchcraft, human hostile behaviour) are more often referred to traditional health care providers (Birdman 2007). Moreover, the acceptability of modern health services is often low due to factors such as poor quality of services, long waiting times and insufficient attention to the patient's specific needs. If patients appear late in the progress of an illness, which is usually the case for many reasons, health workers in modern health services tend to blame the patients for the delay (Tanner and Vlassoff 1998). On the other hand traditional healer are seen as trustworthy, are more likely to give patients a feeling of security, people have been familiar with their practices for generations, and their explanatory models of the illness are better matching (Bugmann 2000) (figure 23).

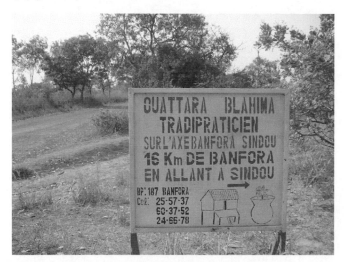

*Figure 23: Traditional medical services in rural south-western Burkina Faso*
*Source: Olaf Müller*

In Burkina Faso, *soumaya* is usually treated at home with a mix of modern and traditional medicine, *djoliban*, if diagnosed, is treated in modern health facilities, while dusukun *yelema* and *kono* are treated through traditional healers (Beiersmann et al. 2007). Similar names and concepts are often found throughout Africa. In Tanzania, *degedege*, representing cerebral malaria, is also believed to be caused by evil spirits and thus treated predominantly by traditional healers (Comoro et al. 2003).

There are large differences between SSA populations on the knowledge and perception of how malaria is transmitted, which has consequences for the uptake of preventive measures. In many endemic areas, while the specific types of fever or malaria symptoms are known, their causes are not associated with the mosquito. In one Gambian study, only 28% of the respondents knew that malaria is transmitted by mosquitoes (Aikins *et al.* 1993). A comparable percentage was found in Tarkwa, Ghana, where only 25% of mothers interviewed said malaria was caused by mosquitoes and a third of the population had no idea at all what causes malaria (Müller 2000). In two other studies assessing the use of malaria prevention measures in households from Malawi and Zimbabwe, 55% of respondents were reported to have identified mosquitoes as the cause of malaria (Vundule and Mharakurwa, 1996). Beside mosquito bites, various other influences are perceived to cause malaria fevers, such as specific food, certain weather or other environmental conditions, and religious explanations (Aikins et al. 1993, Agyepong 1992).

### 2.4.4 Access to health services

Access to modern health services is determined by various factors, which includes geographical access, perceived quality of services, perceived benefit from visiting services, direct (service costs) and indirect (e.g. travel costs, opportunity costs of being away from work) costs, education, and cultural factors (Hutton 2004). In rural Burkina Faso, infant and child mortality was strongly associated with distance to the next health centre (Becher et al. 2004). A large cohort study in young children which was conducted in the same area of Burkina Faso, showed, that fever episodes were mainly self-treated with western drugs or with traditional remedies in the household, and that treatment seeking at formal health services and drug purchase were largely influenced by the distance to such facilities (Müller et al. 2003, Tipke et al. 2009) (figure 24, 25). In rural Burkina Faso, one peripheral health centre – usually staffed by one or two nurses and one midwife, and with an attached pharmacy providing quality-controlled essential drugs – is responsible for a population of about 10.000 scattered over some 7-20

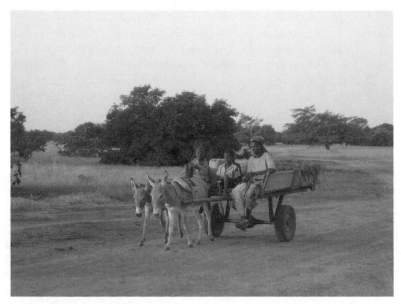

*Figure 24: Traditional transport in rural Burkina Faso*
*Source: Olaf Müller*

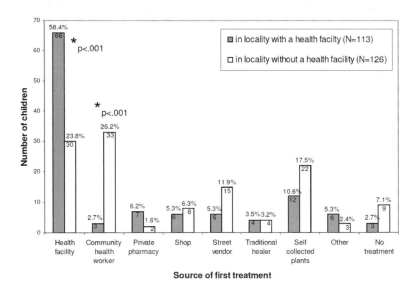

*Figure 25: Antimalarial drug purchase in rural Burkina Faso*
*Source: Tipke et al. (2009)*

villages (Kouyaté et al. 2007) (figure 26, 27). In contrast, traditional healers can be found in nearly every village. Moreover, networks for distributing pharmaceuticals through the illicit market (unlicensed shops, street and market vendors) are widely existing and can often be found in rural areas and villages where no official sources for pharmaceutical products are present (Leonard 2005). Moreover, stocks of medicines in formal health care services have often been reported to be insufficient (Nsimba et al. 1999). In Mali, people living in urban areas were much more likely to visit formal health services in case of fever that were people living in rural areas (Hutton 2004). Public spending is regularly concentrated in urban areas and is thus predominantly benefiting wealthy urban populations (Yates 2009). The costs of formal health services are often, but not always, higher that the costs of traditional health services (Mugisha et al. 2002, Hutton 2004, Beiersmann 2007).

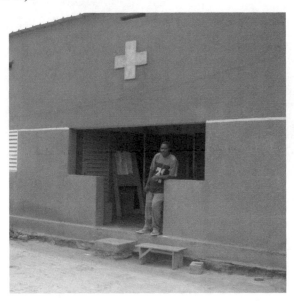

*Figure 26: Peripheral health station in rural Burkina Faso*
*Source: Olaf Müller*

In many countries of SSA, use of modern health facilities is still very low. For example, in the Republic of Congo people visit a modern health facility only once every 7 years (Yates 2009). User fees, which have been widely implemented since the 1980s in all of SSA, had in most occasions clearly a negative effect on access to health care (Mugisha et al. 2002, Hutton 2004, Lagarde & Palmer 2009). There is however some evidence from a few African countries that improved quality in

67

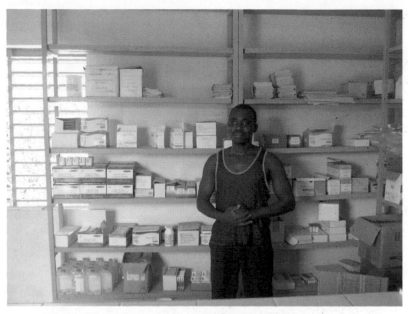

*Figure 27: Pharmacy of a peripheral health station in Burkina Faso*
*Source: Olaf Müller*

creases health service utilisation even under the conditions of continuous user fee charges (Hutton 2004). But overall, user fees decrease access to modern health facilities. They clearly have more profound effects on the poor than on the rich, and tend to delay care and shift people to self-medication and informal forms of care (Hutton 2004, Yates 2009). Furthermore, the idea of exemption schemes for poor people has not been working in practice (Yates 2009). Starting with Uganda in 2001, African countries are now increasingly abolishing user fees (e.g. Zambia, Burundi, Niger, Liberia, Kenya, Senegal, Lesotho, Sudan and Ghana), and this has been accompanied by a significant increase of equitable use of health facilities (Yates 2009). This mainly country-driven movement to increase access to free health care services in SSA, particularly for pregnant women and children younger than five years, is now supported by major bi-lateral and multi-lateral donors including WHO and the World Bank (Yates 2009). But where should the money come from to achieve universal coverage with free quality health services? Ideas include tax-based financing, social health insurance, subsidised community-based health insurance, vouchers, conditional cash transfers, and equity funds (Yates 2009). Besides financing issues, there remains the major challenge of the human resource crisis which has to be addressed in parallel (Narasimhan et al. 2004, Chen et al. 2004, Hongoro & McPake 2004, Omaswa 2008).

Gender dynamics also play a role in access to modern health facilities, particularly in traditional and religious societies. In such societies, women are responsible for the well-being of the majority of household members. At the same time they rarely have the necessary resources at their disposal or the autonomy to make independent decisions. Before seeking care women often have to get permission and/or money from others, like their husband or mother-in-law (Comoro et al. 2003).

Finally, access to quality modern drugs remains a problem in nearly all of the low and middle income countries. The idea of setting up a list with quality-controlled medications that are essential for primary health care in low and middle income countries was part of the *Alma Ata Declaration on Primary Health Care* (PHC) in 1978. The *WHO Model List of Essential Medicines* is now updated every two years since. While 30 years ago, 186 medicines were listed, this number has doubled until today (WHO 2007).

"Essential medicines are those that satisfy the priority health care needs of the population. They are selected with due regard to public health relevance, evidence on efficacy and safety, and comparative cost-effectiveness. Essential medicines are intended to be available within the context of functioning health systems at all times in adequate amounts, in the appropriate dosage forms, with assured quality and adequate information, and at a price the individual and the community can afford. The implementation of the concept of essential medicines is intended to be flexible and adaptable to many different situations; exactly which medicines are regarded as essential remains a national responsibility".

In recent years, increasing numbers of substandard and fake medications were detected in the international markets. It is estimated that more than 10% of the globally traded medicines are counterfeits (Newton et al. 2002). In low and middle income countries, where regulatory and control mechanisms are weak, people are at highest risk to purchase substandard medications (Raufu 2002, Cockburn et al. 2005). Globally it is estimated that around US$70 billion per year are currently earned by the overall trade of substandard and counterfeit drugs (Tipke et al. 2008). After the marketing of the artemisinin-based combination therapy (ACT) in Asia, these costly drugs were found to be largely counterfeit in a number of Southeast Asian countries (Newton et al. 2006a, Hall et al. 2006). In Cambodia, for example, it was shown that fake artesunate was sold by 71% of local drug vendors (Rozendaal 2001).

In SSA, ACTs are currently rolled out in nearly all malaria endemic countries. There is thus great concern that substandard and fake ACTs will enter these African markets (Newman 2010). Available studies from SSA countries have demonstrated already the widespread problem of substandard and fake antimalarial drugs, particularly in the non-public drug sources (Tipke et al. 2008a) (figure 28). In a study from Cameroon for example, 32% of chloroquine, 10% of quinine, and 13% of sulphadoxine/phyrimethamine samples were found to be substandard (Basco 2004). In a study on private pharmacies in Nigeria, 48% of anti-infective drugs, including antimalarials, were found to be of impaired quality (Shakoor 1997). In Burkina Faso, drug quality was recently investigated in a representative sample of modern anti-malarial medications from public and private sources (Tipke et al. 2008b). The sample consisted of chloroquine, pyrimethamine-sulfadoxine, quinine, amodiaquine, artesunate, and arthemeter-lumefantrine. Of 77 drug samples, 32 were found to be of poor quality, 9 had substandard concentrations of the active ingredient, 4 showed poor disintegration, and 1 contained none of the stated active ingredient. The public and the private market contributed 5/47 (10.6%) and 27/30 (90.0%) samples of substandard drugs respectively. A recent report demonstrated similar quality problems with rapid diagnostic tests (RDT) (Newman 2010).

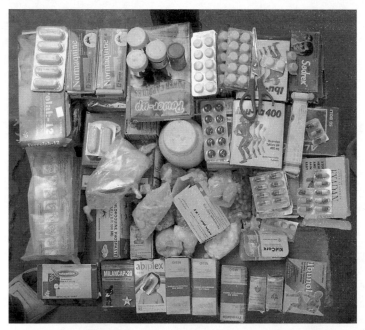

*Figure 28: Diverse drugs sold through unlicensed providers at a local market in north-western Burkina Faso*
*Source: Courtesy Maike Tipke*

## 2.4.5 Malaria risk factors

The risk for malaria infection depends primarily on the transmission intensity in an endemic area. However, within a given endemic situation, the risk for acquiring malaria varies greatly and is influenced by the dominating malaria and vector species, the genetic background of individuals and populations, age in children and pregnancy status in women, weather conditions (season, temperatures, rains), altitude, the availability of preventive measures (e.g. chemoprophylaxis, bed nets and ITNs, vector control), the type of and coverage with malaria first-line treatment, cultural aspects, and socio-economic status (Müller 2000). Various genetic abnormalities have been described to be protective for malaria, ranging from thalassaemia and sickle cell disease to Melanesian ovalocytosis, and from glucose-6-phosphate dehydrogenase (G6PD) deficiency to certain human leukocyte antigens (HLA) types, but results from different studies are often inconsistent (White 2009).

There exist marked differences in malaria parameters between ethnic groups living in the same area. In the central region of Burkina Faso, parasitological data from five cross-sectional surveys showed lower *P. falciparum* prevalence in the Fulani ethnic group for all age groups and lower parasite densities in the Fulani children under 10 years of age as compared to other ethnicities. Moreover, the clinical episodes of malaria were markedly fewer among the Fulani than in the Mossi and Rimaibé (Modiano *et al.* 1996). This was attributed to genetic differences between groups. However, it is also likely that cultural and socio-economic differences between ethnic groups contribute to marked differences in malaria risk, e.g. through differences in exposure or through differences in health seeking behaviour (Brinkmann and Brinkmann, 1991).

In highly endemic areas, malaria parasite rates and densities increase rapidly during infancy (Kitua *et al.* 1996). In all areas of high malaria endemicity, the incidence of clinical malaria is highest in young children (under two years of age) with an average of two to six malaria attacks per year, and both the incidence and the severity of the disease decreases considerably thereafter (Trape *et al.* 1994, Rogier *et al.*1999, Müller et al. 2001). By the age of five years, immunoprotection is reflected by a low rate of malaria attacks despite frequently high parasite densities (Akum Achidi *et al.* 1996).

Malaria is influenced by a large number of environmental factors, which affect its distribution, seasonality and transmission intensity (Snow *et al.* 1999). Highest morbidity and mortality is generally observed in the rainy season, the time when malaria transmission is at its peak, and the number of deaths during this period has been shown to be over threefold higher than in the rest of the year (Jaffar *et al.* 1997, Kynast-Wolf et al. 2005, Hammer et al. 2006, Becher et al. 2008). In a 3-year prospective study of paediatric admissions to the Royal Victoria Hospital in Banjul, The Gambia, 83% of the 1525 children with cerebral malaria were admitted during the extended rainy season from July to December (Brewster and Greenwood, 1993). High levels of parasitemia are also found much more frequently in the rainy season than in the dry season, and anaemia rates are higher the rainy season than in the dry season (Müller et al. 2001, Traoré 2003). The relationship between malaria vector density and the distance of a settlement from a river is an important indicator of malaria transmission. In The Gambia, there was an inverse relationship between the number of mosquitoes in a village and the distance of settlement from the river (Lindsay *et al.* 1993).

It is an epidemiological fact, that low socioeconomic status is strongly associated with poor health outcomes (Marmot et al. 2008). There are comparably few studies regarding the associations between socio-economic status and malaria risk in SSA. In South Africa, poor populations living in mud-walled houses were of a significant higher risk of malaria compared to wealthier households, and sleeping with open windows was identified as an additional risk factor (Coleman et al. 2010). In a large and representative study from the highland areas of Ethiopia, household wealth, living at a higher altitude, and protection with ITNs were protective against malaria, while the intensity of rain was a significant risk factor for malaria (Graves et al. 2009). These findings are supported by the results of a study from the highland areas of Burundi, where the density of *Anopheles* mosquitoes was the main determinant for malaria (Protopopoff et al. 2009).

The epidemiological overlap of HIV and malaria is cause for concern as even a small interaction between the two diseases may be of great public health importance in SSA. Initial studies on this subject from Uganda – one of the countries with the earliest HIV/AIDS epidemics – provided no evidence for measurable large effects (Müller & Moser 1990, Müller et al. 1991). However, further studies from SSA clearly showed that HIV is a risk factor for malaria incidence and severity in pregnant women as well as in adults during the late stage of the HIV/ AIDS disease (Steketee et al. 1996, Verhoeff et al. 1999, Whitworth et al. 2000, French et al. 2001, Korenromp et al. 2005, Hewitt et al. 2006, Abu-Raddad et al. 2006). Among adults in Africa, the association between HIV and malaria does likely result from loss of acquired immunity to malaria. In children the situation is not so clear. In an area of unstable malaria in South Africa HIV was associated with severe malaria in children, but not with parasite density (Grimwade et al. 2003). Another relevant association between HIV/AIDS and malaria in SSA is the risk of HIV infection through contaminated blood transfusions in case of severe malaria anaemia (Hewitt et al. 2006).

Malaria and helminth infections do also overlap geographically to a large extent, and both types of infection induce strong immunomodulation (Hartgers &

Yazdanbakhsh 2006). Analyses of clinical interactions between helminth and malaria coinfection have so far produced conflicting results; while some studies have documented increased malaria morbidity associated with coinfection, other have shown the opposite (Druilhe et al. 2005, Brutus et al. 2006). However, helminth infections seem to protect from more severe manifestations of malaria (Specht & Hoerauf 2007). If helminth coinfection allows for higher malaria parasitaemia at lower levels of disease severity, it is not clear what this means for ongoing mass treatment programs of helminths in SSA (Specht & Hoerauf 2007).

Malnutrition remains the major risk factor for mortality in young children of SSA, but data on associations of public health importance between malaria and malnutrition are inconclusive (Müller et al. 2002, Müller et al. 2003, Müller & Krawinkel 2005, Müller & Becher 2006). Protein energy malnutrition (PEM) was partly shown to be protective and partly to be a risk factor (Müller et al. 2002). Such effects could be of large public health importance as a great proportion of young children in SSA are at risk for both malaria and malnutrition (Müller & Krawinkel 2005). Moreover, controlled trials on the effects of micronutrient supplementation with vitamin A or zinc on malaria provided conflicting results (Müller et al. 2001, Müller et al. 2002). A large study investigating the effects of zinc supplementation on malaria morbidity has shown no differences between intervention and control group (Müller et al. 2001). There is also an ongoing discussion regarding the benefits and risks of iron supplementation in areas of malaria endemicity. More recent data are now strongly supporting a positive association between iron supplementation and malaria incidence in SSA areas of malaria, which has important policy implications (Sazawal et al. 2006).

### 2.4.6 Epidemiological prototypes

Based on the characteristics of an endemic area, different epidemiological prototypes can be defined (Gilles 1993). The *African savannah malaria type* clearly is the most important with regard to transmission intensity and morbidity and mortality (figure 29). Here, the EIR often reaches several hundred infective bites per person per year, which is accompanied by a high burden of malaria in young children and in pregnant women (Müller et al. 2001). Moreover, the populations in these areas are regularly very poor and have little access to functioning health services (Müller et al. 2003). The characteristics of this prototype are demonstrated by the situation in the research zone of the *Centre de Recherche en Santé de Nouna* (CRSN) in the Kossi Province in north-western Burkina Faso (Sié et al. 2010). In such areas, the prevalence of *P. falciparum* infection, the corresponding spleen rates, and falciparum malaria incidence are very high with a clear peak towards the end of the rainy season and with malaria being the main cause of fever in young children (figure 30-33). In *African savannah*, mortality typically peaks during infancy with most cases of malaria-attributed deaths occurring during the second half of infancy, when the passively acquired immunity is waning rapidly, as shown by the pattern of cause-specific mortality determined by verbal autopsy diagnosis in the HDSS of the CRSN in Burkina Faso (table 4).

Another prototype of malaria epidemiology is the type of *forest-related malaria*, which is associated to exploitation of forests by human populations such as hunters, gold and gem miners, inhabitants of new settlements and indigenous populations. These are then exposed to vector populations adapted to breeding sites in the forest, which can't easily be controlled. Quantitatively, this prototype is not playing a major role in SSA until today.

The *desert fringe and highland fringe prototype* of malaria epidemiology affects mainly nomadic populations or minority groups living in such areas. However, also large populations living in the highland areas of countries such as Ethiopia, Kenya, Madagascar, Zimbabwe and in the fringe areas of the Sahel Zone and southern Africa are affected. Here, long dry seasons or high altitude (malaria transmission is possible up to 2.000 – 2.500 m) coupled with low population density and frequent movements of populations make them susceptible to epidemics with high morbidity and mortality due to low immunity of the populations. Such epidemics are often triggered by changing weather conditions and large population movements. Moreover, increasing mobility of local populations results in people with low immunity frequently visiting places of higher transmission intensity and thus contracting severe malaria. In Africa, this prototype will become increasingly important in the future due to larger populations, increasing mobility and the dynamics of global warming (Hay et al. 2004).

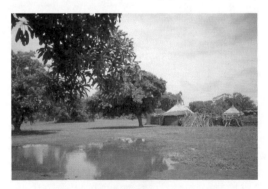

*Figure 29: African savannah area in rural north-western Burkina Faso*
*Source: Olaf Müller*

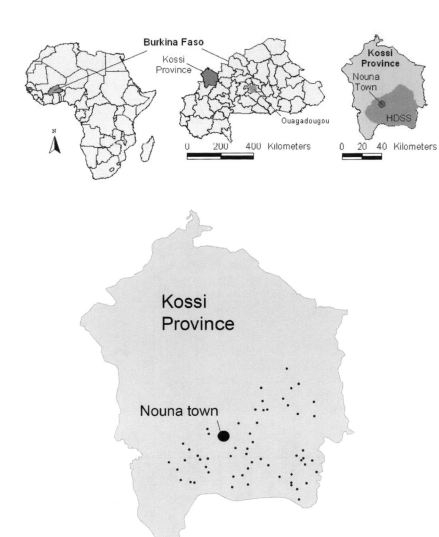

*Figure 30: Study zone of the Centre de Recherche en Santé de Nouna (CRSN)*
*Source: Traoré (2003)*

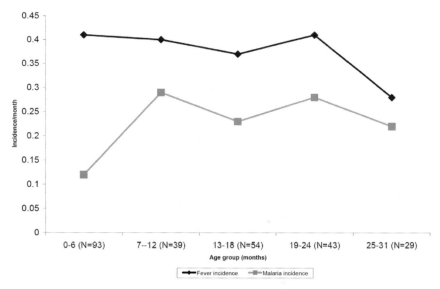

*Figure 31: Fever and falciparum malaria incidence in young children of Burkina Faso*
*Source: Traoré (2003)*

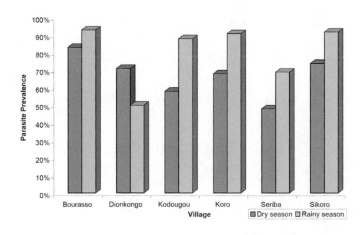

*Figure 32: P. falciparum prevalence in young children of six villages in Burkina Faso*
*Source: Traoré (2003)*

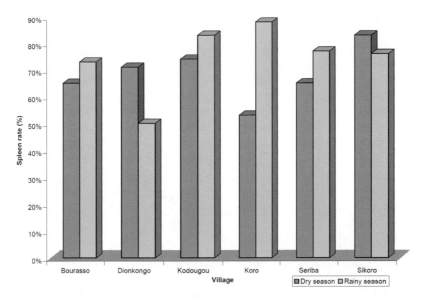

*Figure 33: Spleen rates in young children of six villages in Burkina Faso*
*Source: Traoré (2003)*

| Age (months) | Cause of deaths | | | | | |
|---|---|---|---|---|---|---|
| | MAL | ARI | GE | Others | Missing | Total |
| 0-6 | 9 | 4 | 4 | 12 | 1 | 30 |
| 7-12 | 11 | 1 | 4 | 2 | 13 | 31 |
| 13-18 | 9 | 2 | 3 | 2 | 3 | 19 |
| 19-24 | 6 | 1 | 9 | 2 | 1 | 19 |
| 25-36 | 7 | 1 | 3 | 2 | 6 | 19 |
| Total | 42 | 9 | 23 | 20 | 24 | 118 |

MAL=malaria; ARI=acute respiratory infection; GE=gastroenteritis

*Table 4: Causes of death by age group in young children of rural Burkina Faso*
*Source: Traoré (2003)*

With increasing urbanisation, the *prototype of urban malaria* becomes more and more important in SSA (figure 34). Although breeding conditions are usually not good for the malaria vectors in the inner city areas, the surrounding suburban and slum areas often provide sufficient breeding places to support ongoing malaria transmission. This may mainly play a role during the rainy season but could also be changed to perennial transmission due to existing permanent water bodies such as dam projects. In Ethiopia, it has been shown that the establishment of micro-dams was associated with a significant increase in malaria incidence (Ghebreyesus et al. 1999). In general, transmission intensity tends to be lower in urban areas as compared to the surrounding rural areas and access to health services is usually much better in the cities (Wang et al. 2005, Wang et al. 2006). Malaria-specific mortality was recently shown to be much lower in urban compared to rural areas in Burkina Faso (Ramroth et al. 2009).

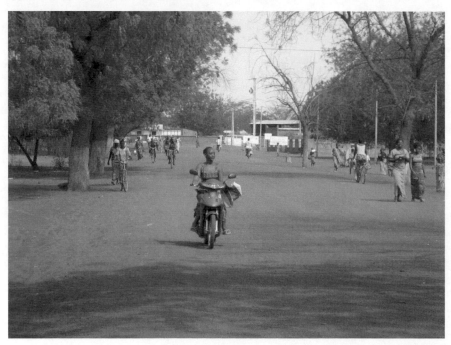

*Figure 34: Semi-urban area in Burkina Faso (Nouna town)*
*Source: Olaf Müller*

Another important prototype in Africa is the *agricultural development type* with its various consequences on malaria. For example, dam and irrigation projects may convert areas of seasonal malaria transmission into areas of perennial transmission due to the establishment of permanent breeding places. On the other hand, such development projects often lead to an improved socio-economic situation of the population, which enables them to live in better houses, to sleep under mosquito nets, and to have better access to malaria prophylaxis and treatment (figure 35). The consequence of such a complex change can be a much reduced malaria burden which was called "paddies paradox" (Ijumba & Lindsay 2001). Moreover, development projects are often associated with urbanisation and more intense malaria control due to the importance of certain industries. Finally, clearing of forests for the establishment of new settlers can be associated with changes in the dominating malaria vectors which may have dramatic consequences in case of the establishment of *An. gambiae* and *An. funestus,* sometimes even being compounded by lower immunity of the newly established population.

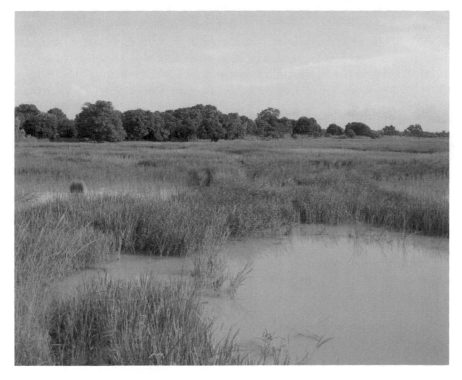

*Figure 35: Rice fields in north-western Burkina Faso*
*Source: Olaf Müller*

Other prototypes of malaria epidemiology which play a certain role in SSA are the *coastal and marshland type* (associated with lower transmission intensity due to environmental and socio-economic characteristics, and with brackish water breeding vectors such as *An. melas* in West Africa and *An. merus* in East Africa, which have a lower vectorial capacity), and the epidemiological *type associated with socio-political disturbances* (associated with increased morbidity and mortality due to displacement of populations and general disruption of health services) (Gilles 1993).

## 2.5 Resistance

### 2.5.1 Resistance to antimalarials

Microorganisms usually become resistant to every antimicrobial agent that is used on a large scale, and this also applies to the malaria parasites (White 2004, Talisuna et al. 2004). However, there are considerable differences between the different antimalarials regarding the speed of resistance development (Wongsrichanalai et al. 2002) (table 5). The earliest reports of resistance to an antimalarial dates back to 1910 for quinine (Talisuna et al. 2004). However, this drug – which has been used successfully for 350 years – is still among the most effective antimalarials in the world. The main reason for this is probably the relatively low drug pressure over time due to low access and its annoying side effects, coupled with the short half-life of quinine, which prevents longer periods of sub-therapeutic drug concentrations in the blood (Meshnick 1997).

| Antimalarial drug | Introduced | First reported resistance | Difference (years) |
|---|---|---|---|
| Quinine | 1632 | 1910 | 278 |
| Chloroquine | 1945 | 1957 | 12 |
| Proguanil | 1948 | 1949 | 1 |
| Sulfadoxine-pyrimethamine | 1967 | 1967 | 0 |
| Mefloquine | 1977 | 1982 | 5 |
| Artesunate* | 1977 | 2007 | 30 |
| Atovaquone | 1996 | 1996 | 0 |
| *Dondorp et al. 2009 | | | |

*Table 5: Dates of introduction and first reports of antimalarial drug resistance*

Resistance to the early antimalarials proguanil and pyrimethamine already dates back some 50 years, and first resistance to chloroquine developed initially and independently in Thailand in 1957 and in South America in 1959 (Warrell 1993). As a result of population movement from Asia, chloroquine resistance arrived at the coast of East Africa towards the end of the 1970s from where it has spread continuously inland (Kean 1979, Wernsdorfer 1994, Müller et al. 1996, Talisuna et al. 2004). As a consequence, malaria morbidity and mortality rates were increasing in many parts of SSA but mainly in East and South Africa (Trapé et al. 2001, Korenromp 2003). However, chloroquine resistance was more recently also observed to rapidly spread in West Africa, as exemplified by a number of studies in north-western Burkina Faso (Müller et al. 2003, Meissner et al. 2005, Meissner et al. 2006, Meissner et al. 2008). The spread of resistance was more marked in urban as compared to rural areas (Danquah et al. 2010).

As a consequence of the chloroquine resistance development, the policy for first-line treatment of fever and malaria cases was subsequently changed in all malaria endemic African countries, starting with the KwaZulu-Natal province in South Africa in 1988 and in Malawi in 1993 (Talisuna et al. 2004). Such a change of policy is usually informed by surveillance of parasite susceptibility and needs to be planned and implemented very carefully (Hastings et al. 2007). Countries initially changed from chloroquine to pyrimethamine-sulfadoxine or amodiaquine, which however did not last long before a further change became necessary. The more rapid resistance development against antifolates compared to the 4-aminoquinolines is likely linked to the smaller number of genetic mutations needed (Hastings et al. 2002). As chloroquine resistance is linked to multiple mutations in PFCRT, a protein that functions as a transporter in the *P. falciparum* parasite's digestive vacuole membrane, the development and spread of chloroquine resistance can also be monitored using CRT as a molecular marker (Wellems & Plowe 2001, Sidhu et al. 2002, Wongsrichanalai et al. 2002). Interestingly, it has become documented that antimalarials such as chloroquine regain their efficacy after having not been used for several years (Laufer et al. 2006). This observation is supported by decreasing CRT mutation prevalence over the dry season in the Nouna study area in Burkina Faso and points to a biological advantage of the wild type parasites (Müller, unpublished).

The gold standard for the assessment of *P. falciparum* susceptibility is the *in vivo* therapeutic response to antimalarials (Wongsrichanalai et al. 2002). *In vivo* sensitivity to drugs was originally defined by WHO as parasite clearance. Since 1996, there exist modified WHO protocols, which are mainly based on clinical outcomes. Such protocols are more useful in areas of intense transmission as in most of SSA (Wongsrichanalai et al. 2002, WHO 2003) (table 6). Discrimination between recrudescence and reinfection is usually achieved by molecular methods

(WHO 2003). *In vivo* assessment of *P. falciparum* susceptibility should be undertaken in patients with low immunity, which in areas of high transmission intensity usually are young children, as more potent immune responses increase the efficacy of chemotherapy. The susceptibility of *P. falciparum* against antimalarial drugs can also be investigated by assays measuring the inhibition of parasite development *in vitro*, but results do not necessarily correspond to *in vivo* findings due to the role of immunity and other host factors. Finally, pharmacokinetic information is needed to differentiate between true resistance and inadequate drug concentrations.

| Classification | Definition |
| --- | --- |
| *Original classification* | |
| S (sensitive) | Reduction to <25% of initial parasitaemia on day 2 with smears negative for malaria from day 7 to the end of follow-up (usually 28 days) |
| RI response | Initial clearance of parasitaemia, a negative smear on day 7, followed by recrudescence afterwards |
| RII response | Initial clearance or substantial reduction of parasitaemia (<25% of the initial count on day 2) but with persistence or recrudescence of parasitaemia during days 4-7 |
| RIII response | No significant reduction of parasitaemia |
| | |
| *Modified classification* | |
| Early Treatment failure (ETF) | Development of danger signs or severe malaria in the presence of parasitaemia during the first 3 days of follow-up; parasitaemia on day 2 higher than day 0; parasitaemia on day 3 with fever; parasitaemia on day 3 > 25% of count on day 0 |
| Late Clinical Failure (LCF) | Development of danger signs or severe malaria in the presence of parasitaemia between day 4 and end of follow-up; presence of parasitaemia with fever between day 4 and end of follow-up |

| Late Parasitological Failure (LPF) | Presence of parasitaemia on any day from day 7 until end of follow-up |
|---|---|
| Adequate Clinical and | Absence of parasitaemia at the end of follow-up without |
| Parasitological Response (ACPR) | previously meeting any of the criteria of ETF, LCF or LPF |

*Table 6: Classification of in vivo antimalarial drug sensitivity*

The factors responsible for the emergence and spread of malaria parasite resistance are not fully understood, but drug selective pressure, drug half-life and malaria transmission intensity are likely the most important determinants (White & Pongtavornpinyo 2003, Talisuna et al. 2004). Today, combination therapy has become the new paradigm in malaria treatment with the main objective to avert or at least delay resistance development (White et al. 1999, White 2004, Greenwood 2005). Artemisinin-based combination therapy (ACT) has evolved as the gold standard of malaria combination therapy, with a number of safe and effective regimens available (Olliaro & Wells 2009). This development was very much pushed by the World Health Organisation despite the availability of cheap alternatives (such as amodiaquine-sulfadoxine-pyrimethamine), which could have served as an intermediate step before moving to ACT in SSA (Kouyaté et al. 2007).

Artemisinin derivates – while killing the young intraerythrocytic parasites –rapidly reduce the parasite biomass including gametocytes, which results in rapid clinical relief and also in reduction of resistant and non-resistant parasite transmission (White 2008, White 2009). The efficacy of such regimes has been demonstrated under programme conditions in South-East Asia, where the combination of artesunate-mefloquine has halted the development of mefloquine resistance and also reduced the falciparum malaria burden (Price et al. 1996, Nosten et al. 2000). However, it is currently not clear whether the same results can be obtained in SSA, where transmission intensity is much higher. As most antimalarials combined with the artemisinins have a much longer half-life, new infections will get exposed to sub-therapeutic blood levels of these drugs with the possibility of subsequent resistance development (Talisuna et al. 2004). Until very recently, ACTs were frequently provided as co-blisters in national programmes which enabled the patient to individually decide if he likes to take either components or only one of them. It has been observed in rural Burkina Faso that patients were selectively only taking the artesunate tablets as they did not like the amodiaquine component of the amodiaquine-artesunate combination (Müller et al. 2009a). Such problems with compliance would certainly have an impact on resistance development and it is thus promising that most programmes now switch to fixed-dose ACT regimens.

Global malaria control today rests on the sustained efficacy of a single class of drugs, the artemisinins (WHO 2008b). It has thus become very worrying, that there are first reports about *in vivo* resistance development against artemisinins from South-East Asia (Dondorp et al. 2009). Although it is currently not clear what exactly is happening and what are the main determinants for such development, it is a fact that there are no good alternatives to artemisinin derivates in the late pipeline of drug development (Olliaro & Wells 2009). In this regard, it has recently been proposed to add further drugs (such as methylene blue) to ACTs to better protect the artemisinin component and to further reduce gametocytaemia (Müller et al. 2009a).

## 2.5.2 Resistance to insecticides

Although there are more insecticides available for malaria control as it has been the case some 50 years ago, the chemical arsenal remains rather limited (Kelly-Hope et al. 2008). For indoor residual spraying (IRS), four insecticide classes are available today – carbamates, organophosphates, organochlorines, and pyrethroids. ITNs but not IRS is currently the main strategy for malaria prevention in most of SSA (Greenwood et al. 2005). However, for the ITN intervention only one insecticide class – the pyrethroids – is approved by the WHO Pesticides Evaluation Scheme (WHOPES).

During the time of the Malaria Eradication Programme of the 1950s and 60s, resistance of *Anopheles* mosquitoes against DDT has already been recorded in SSA (Müller 2000). DDT resistance can be due either to a specific detoxification mechanism (glutathione-S-transferase) or to a modification of the target site. DDT and pyrethroids have the same target in the voltage-gated sodium channel (Ranson et al. 2010). Point mutations at this target cause knock down resistance (*kdr*). This type of resistance, governed by the *kdr* gene, reduces both the knockdown and lethal effects of DDT and has been shown to induce a cross-resistance to pyrethroids. Two alternative amino acid substitutions at the same position (1014) confer resistance, one being termed *kdr west* and the other *kdr east* (Ranson et al. 2010). The link between the *kdr* genotype and pyrethroid resistance phenotype is clear, but might only explain a portion of the heritable variation in resistance (Donnelly et al. 2009). Beside target site resistance, metabolic, cuticular and behavioural resistance also play important roles in the response of mosquitoes to the insecticides (Ranson et al. 2010).

Since the 1970s, pyrethroids have been extensively used in urban areas (coils and aerosols) as well as for agricultural purposes (particularly cotton) in rural areas of SSA (figure 36). As a consequence, the first case of pyrethroid resistance in *An. gambiae s.l.* was recorded in Ivory Coast (Chandre et al. 1999, Ranson et al. 2010), and *kdr* is now widespread in SSA (Etang et al. 2006, Donnelly et al. 2009). Based on bioassay results, *kdr* resistance phenotype and genotype were found to be correlated in *Anopheles gambiae* populations of SSA (Ranson et al. 2000, Ranson et al. 2010). However, whether and to which degree *kdr* undermines the effectiveness of insecticide-treated materials (ITM) in areas of high prevalence and what are the determinants of such a development is still unclear. While studies in Ivory Coast and Burkina Faso had shown that ITM remained effective despite high frequency of *kdr* (Donnelly et al. 2009), in Benin the efficacy of ITM was negatively associated with the presence of high level *kdr* resistance in *An. gambiae* populations (N'Guessan et al. 2007). Finally, in the Nouna area of north-western Burkina Faso no differences were observed in the susceptibility of *Anopheles* mosquitoes to pyrethroids between an urban area and villages with and without cotton agriculture (Schroer et al. unpublished) (figure 37).

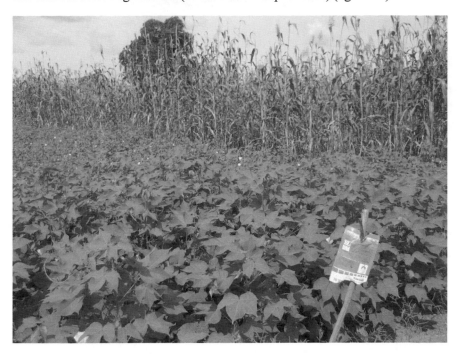

*Figure 36: Cotton agriculture in north-western Burkina Faso with extensive use of pyrethroid insecticides*
*Source: Olaf Müller*

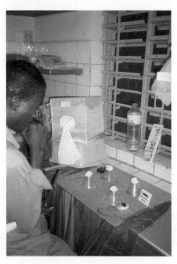

*Figure 37: Phenotypical testing of ITNs for pyrethroid resistance in Burkina Faso*
*Source: Olaf Müller*

As with antimalarial drugs, there is clearly an ongoing need for development of new insecticides, an area which is mainly driven by the agricultural sector. However, there are some promising developments, such as improved formulations of existing insecticides, successful trials of ITNs with alternative insecticides such as carbamates and organophosphates, adding pyrethroid-treated plastic sheeting to other vector control interventions, or even combinations of pyrethroids and entomopathogenic fungi (Kelly-Hope et al. 2008, Chandre et al. 2010, Farenhorst et al. 2010). Moreover, the importance of insecticide resistance monitoring and integrated vector management has become more obvious in the recent past (Kelly-Hope et al. 2008). A clear prerequisite for this would be the development of local entomological capacity in African countries.

## 2.6 Malaria and development

Malaria is a disease of poverty (Müller 2004). There is a strong relation between the burden of malaria and the socio-economic status of respective countries. In 1995, the average gross domestic product (GDP) per head was 1.526 US$ in malaria endemic countries as compared to 8.268 US$ in neighbouring countries where malaria was eliminated as a public health problem (Sachs & Malaney 2002). Countries endemic for malaria do not only demonstrate a lower GDP when compared to non endemic countries, their economy also grows much slower. The average increase in GDP per head over the period 1965 until 1990 was only 0.4% per year in endemic as compared to 2.3% in non endemic countries (Sachs & Malaney 2002).

Poverty is usually associated with poor hygiene and poor housing conditions, but also with lack of money and information regarding malaria treatment and prevention (Gallup & Sachs 2001). Whereas in countries outside Africa malaria is mainly a problem of ethnic minority populations in remote areas, in most of SSA it is still a problem of the general populations (Snow et al. 1999). Malaria thus remains a major contributor to the vicious circle of poverty and ill-health in SSA. The elimination of malaria in many industrialised countries between 1930 and 1950 was primarily the result of major socio-economic development coupled with targeted malaria control activities (Sachs & Malaney 2002).

The economic costs of malaria include its effects on the individual, the household, the community, and the economic development (Breman et al. 2006). Malaria causes high direct and indirect household costs. This includes costs for preventive and curative measures, costs for transport to health services, costs for not being able to work, and costs related to disability and death (Nur 1993). These costs are relatively high for the households with the lowest income, who in turn carry the highest malaria burden (Gallup & Sachs 2001). Such effects vary with the age distribution of malaria-attributed morbidity and mortality in different endemic regions. In Africa, where disease and death is concentrated among young children, the effects are different from other areas where disease and deaths occur mainly among the breadwinners or primary caretakers of families (Breman et al. 2006). Being the most prevalent disease in the rural areas of Africa, malaria produces much loss of productivity during the rainy seasons, when there is a peak demand for agricultural work (Sauerborn et al. 1996). It is common to find the parameter of seven days of work lost to disability per bout of malaria (Over 1992). It has been estimated that the prevention and treatment of malaria makes up for some 10% of the expenses of an average household in SSA and around 40% of the total spending on public health in Africa (Kager 2002).

In countries with high malaria endemicity, a large proportion of the childhood mortality is typically attributed to malaria (Hammer et al. 2006). The degree of childhood mortality remains one of the main determinants for continuously high fertility rates in SSA beside the education of the mother, the socio-economic status of the household and the availability of modern family planning methods (Müller & Jahn 2009). In such populations, children remain the main social security net for the majority of the still rural populations living on subsistence agriculture (Müller 2004).

Other problems malaria causes are related to the educational sector which is also key for the overall development of societies. Households with many children can't invest much into the education of the individual child. Moreover, children are often absent from school because they have fallen ill to malaria. Thus, a significant impairment of children's education in endemic regions has early been attributed to malaria (Macdonald 1950). The long-term effects of repeated and sometimes severe malaria episodes on the neuro-cognitive development of children living in malaria endemic regions are associated with poor performance at school and afterwards and are thus likely to have serious long-term consequences for the development of such societies (Gallup & Sachs 2001).

The rather low investment of private enterprises in malaria endemic countries can be considered as one of the major barriers to the development of such countries and regions. Investors avoid malaria endemic countries fearing for the health of themselves and their staff. This can be illustrated by an example from Mozambique, where an English mine company has recently invested 1.4 billion US$. Within two years, some 7,000 staff had fallen ill to malaria and 13 expatriate staff died because of this disease (Gallup & Sachs 2001). Moreover, tourism as one of the major income resources of low and middle income countries is highly affected by the malaria risk (Sachs & Malaney 2002).

Malaria always had a significant influence on the global relations between countries. While it may even have been protective for African populations during the time of colonialism, today it is clearly a major impediment for development (Gallup & Sachs 2001). This is also documented by the strong acceleration of socio-economic development in the countries of southern Europe some 50 years ago, when malaria elimination was followed by major investments of private industry (Gallup & Sachs 2001).

# Chapter 3. Control and elimination of malaria in Africa

## 3.1 Introduction

There are two major short-term and one long-term strategy in the battle against malaria. The first short-term strategy addresses the parasite in the human host through case management with different antimalarial drugs and supportive treatments, while the second one targets the *Anopheles* vector through different vector control approaches ranging from the application of insecticides against the mosquitoes and/or their larvae to environmental modification. In addition, there are a number of older (e.g. mosquito repellents) or newer (e.g. vaccines) tools. There is now an overall agreement in the malaria community, that control programmes need to implement a comprehensive mix of the available and locally appropriate tools (Greenwood et al. 2005, Breman et al. 2006). In countries which move from a control to an elimination approach, the strategy needs to be adapted with a strong emphasis on surveillance (WHO 2009b). Clearly, overall development associated with decreasing poverty, better education, more protective housing, enforced environmental control of breeding sites and in particular improved preventive and curative health services is the most promising long-term strategy and will ultimately lead to control and finally elimination in most endemic areas (figure 38).

## 3.2 Tools and strategies for control and elimination

### 3.2.1 Case management in health facilities

The first element of the *Global Malaria Control Strategy* – to provide early diagnosis and prompt treatment – remains the most important one of the four technical elements (WHO 1993a). For the last half century case management of uncomplicated malaria was equivalent to syndromic treatment of fever cases in SSA (Müller 2000). However, the rapid increase of chloroquine resistance in recent years let to universal changes to alternative malaria first-line treatments, which are now ACT in the whole of SSA (WHO 2009b). Given the still significantly higher costs of ACT compared to former chloroquine or sulfadoxine-pyrimeth-

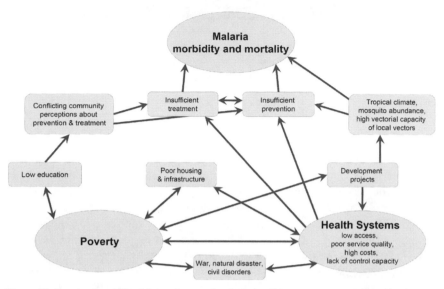

*Figure 38: Proximal and distal determinants of malaria in Africa*

amine monotherapies and the still limited production capacity, malaria case management based on laboratory diagnosis of the parasites has been considered to be more cost-effective and to also contribute to a delay in resistance development against artemisinin compounds (Greenwood et al. 2005). Laboratory-based diagnosis is not only perceived as beneficial to avoid overtreatment of non-malaria cases with ACT but also to help diagnose and to treat correctly fever cases of alternative causes (Björkman & Martensson 2010). Given the ongoing successes of the RBM activities in many regions (see 3.4.4), the malaria-attributable fraction of fever cases is likely to diminish further making diagnosis-based fever treatment strategies even more important. As a consequence, WHO now generally recommends prompt parasitological confirmation of diagnoses in all patients suspected of malaria before treatment is started (Zarocostas 2010, Björkman & Martensson 2010).

Recent estimates point to less than 10 percent of suspected malaria cases having received a parasitological diagnosis in Africa (WHO 2008b). Until recently, laboratory diagnosis of malaria was based on malaria blood slides and light microscopy (Perkins & Bell 2008) (figure 39, 40). However, access to and the quality of microscopic diagnosis in the health services of SSA remains rather limited. RDTs, which are easy to handle even by non-technicians, have been considered to be an alternative (Greenwood et al. 2005). RDTs are cheaper than ACT and thus likely to be cost-effective, but only if the diagnoses are respected by the health workers (Perkins & Bell 2008, Anonymous 2010a). In a recently conducted large randomised controlled trial (RCT) in Ghana, the use of RDTs was not more effective than microscopy but significantly more effective than clinical diagnosis in reducing overprescription of antimalarials (Ansah et al. 2010). However, studies in many African countries including Burkina Faso have shown that laboratory diagnosis does not necessarily change the prescription behaviour and may even be harmful (Reyburn et al. 2007, Hamer et al. 2007, Pfeiffer et al. 2008, Skarbinski et al. 2009, Bisoffi et al. 2009, Chinkhumba et al. 2010). Although RDTs have high sensitivity and specificity for falciparum malaria, they still carry the risk of false positive and false negative diagnosis, particularly at low parasite densities, and they are costly (Greenwood et al. 2005, Björkman & Martensson 2010). Moreover, there are considerable differences between the test characteristics and their performance under real life conditions (WHO 2008a, WHO 2009a, Chinkhumba et al. 2010). Currently a lot of research is going on which looks at the feasibility, safety, cost-efficacy and effectiveness of RDTs in SSA, and initial results are promising (Msellem et al. 2009, Ssekabira et al. 2008, Björkman & Martensson 2010).

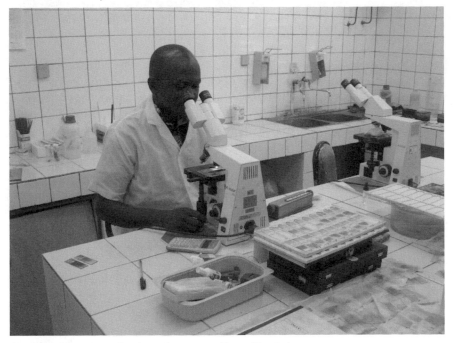

*Figure 39: Microscopical malaria diagnosis in Nouna Hospital*
*Source: Olaf Müller*

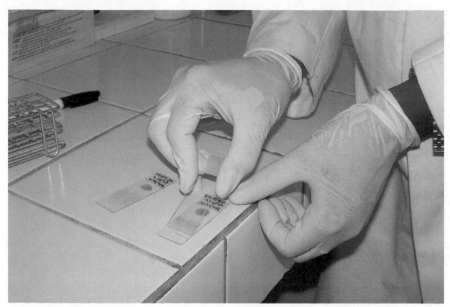

*Figure 40: Preparation of blood slides for malaria diagnosis in Burkina Faso*
*Source: Olaf Müller*

Available antimalarial compounds include the arylaminoalcohols (e. g. quinine, mefloquine), 4-aminoquinolines (e. g. chloroquine, amodiaquine), sulfones and sulfonamides (e. g. sulfadoxine), biguanides and related substances (e. g. proguanil, pyrimethamine), 8-aminoquinolines (e. g. primaquine), antibiotics (e. g. tetracyclines, clindamycin), naphthoquinones (atovaquone), and peroxide antimalarials (e. g. artemisinin, artemether) (Müller 2000).

Treating malaria with a combination of effective drugs with different mechanisms has become a new paradigm in malaria control, with the particular aim to delay and possibly reverse the development of drug resistance (White et al. 1999, Nosten and Brasseur 2002). In particular artemisinin drugs in combination with a variety of partner drugs have proved highly effective in a number of field trials (International Artemisinin Study Group 2002, Abacassamo et al. 2004, Piola et al. 2005, Mutabingwa et al. 2005, Sutherland et al. 2005, Ratcliff et al. 2007). In addition to registered ACTs, two more and promising ACTs – dihydroartemisinin-piperaquine (Tran et al. 2004, Smithuis et al. 2006, Zwang et al. 2009) and artesunate-pyronaridine (Tshefu et al. 2010) – have already successfully past phase II/III trials and are close to registration. Although the costs for artemisinin-based combination therapy (ACT) remain significantly higher than the costs for chloroquine and pyrimethamine-sulfadoxine regimens, nearly all African countries have already switched their antimalarial first line treatment policy to ACT (WHO 2009). Today, there are also a number of fixed-dose ACT regimens on the market, but arthemeter-lumefantrine and artesunate-amodiaquine are those mainly used in malaria control programmes in SSA. However, the availability of paediatric formulations of antimalarials remains very limited. It is thus promising, that a paediatric formulation of artemether-lumefantrine (a dispersible tablet) has recently been developed for infants (Abdulla et al. 2008a).

It is important to provide treatment as fixed-dose regimens to not risk the development of resistance against the artemisinins (Anonymous 2009a). It has been shown for example in Burkina Faso that the provision of artesunate-amodiaquine as separate blister tablets resulted in de facto artesunate monotherapy due to frequent side effects of amodiaquine in this population (Müller et al. 2009a). There is now sufficient evidence that ACT combinations improve efficacy without increasing toxicity, but cure rates vary widely and mainly depend on the level of resistance against the partner drug. However, some alternative combinations such as amodiaquine-pyrimethamine/sulfadoxine and amodiaquine-methylene blue were shown to be at least equally effective when compared to ACT in certain African populations (Zongo et al. 2007, Zoungrana et al. 2008).

WHO currently recommends the following combination regimens (WHO 2009b):

1. artemether/lumefantrine
2. dihydroartemisinin-pipcraquine
3. artesunate-amodiaquine (in areas where the cure rate of amodiaquine monotherapy is greater than 80%)
4. artesunate-mefloquine (insufficient safety data to recommend its use in Africa)
5. artesunate-sulfadoxine/pyrimethamine (in areas where the cure rate of sulfadoxine/pyrimethamine is greater than 80%)
6. amodiaquine-sulfadoxine/pyrimethamine (may be considered as an interim option where ACTs cannot be made available, provided that efficacy of both is high)
7. chloroquine-primaquine (only for vivax malaria in areas where chloroquine has remained effective)
8. atovaquone-proguanil (only for travellers)

Artemisinin and related compounds are a structurally new group of antimalarial drugs, which have been isolated in China in 1972 from the plant *Artemesia annua*. Artemisinin was initially formulated in China in both oil and water for intramuscular injections and as tablets and suppositories (Meshnik et al. 1996). More potent artemisinin derivates are artesunate and artemether, with sodium artesunate being applicable for intravenous administration. No major clinical toxicity has been reported in humans until today, and artemisinin derivates are the most rapidly acting of all existing antimalarial drugs (Hien and White 1993, De Vries and Dien 1996). As artemisinin compounds have been shown to exhibit a pronounced effect on gametocytes, they may also contribute to reductions of malaria transmission levels (Price et al. 1996, von Seidlein et al. 1998). Unfortunately and based on the still frequent use of monotherapies, resistance against artemisinin compounds has recently started to emerge in South-East Asia (Noedl et al. 2008). There is thus a clear need to preserve the efficacy of the artemisinin compounds through avoidance of monotherapies and possibly through adding other drugs with better matching pharmacokinetic properties and less potential for resistance development to existing ACTs, such as methylene blue (Müller et al. 2009a). Methylene blue has the further advantage to act against both the young and the old gametocytes, with the promise to further reduce transmission (Coulibaly et al. 2009). Although the global antimalarial drug portfolio is quite good in these days, most potential alternatives to artemisinin compounds are still in a very early state of development and a true emergence of wide-spread artemisinin resistance would be a public health disaster comparable to the history of chloroquine resistance development (Ollario & Wells 2009).

The combination of the new hydroxynaphthoquinone atovaquone and proguanil (Malarone[R]) is now also widely registered for treatment and prevention (Hudson 1993, Looareesuwan et al. 1996, Radloff et al. 1996, de Alencar et al. 1997, Lell et al. 1998). However, the large-scale application of this drug in Africa is unlikely due to the high prize and the potential for rapid resistance development (Bloland et al. 1997).

Treatment options for pregnant women remain limited, mainly due to uncertainties regarding the safety of artemisinin drugs in the first trimester. A currently available alternative is the combination of quinine and clindamycin, which is however costly (Chico & Chandramohan 2010). The malaria efficacy of azithromycin has first been identified in an earlier epidemiological study in The Gambia (Sadiq et al. 1995), and azithromycin with quinine as well as azithromycin with chloroquine are promising combinations currently under investigation for to be given in any trimester (Chico & Chandramohan 2010).

The community effectiveness of an intervention under real life conditions is regularly much lower than the efficacy measured in randomised controlled trials (Krause & Sauerborn 2000). The reasons for this are obvious shortcomings within the health systems. Such system problems thus regularly reduce the expected benefits of otherwise very promising interventions (Lengeler & Snow 1996). Causes are many, ranging from limited geographical availability of health services, lack of money for transport and services, low acceptability and quality of services, and suboptimal sensitivity and specificity of diagnostics to the many factors associated with poor patient adherence. The combined effect of this is usually high and has a major impact on the expected impact of interventions at programme level. Figure 41 estimates the resulting community effectiveness of a highly efficacious ACT when delivered in a poorly functioning health system in SSA (based on data from studies conducted in the Nouna Health District in Burkina Faso).

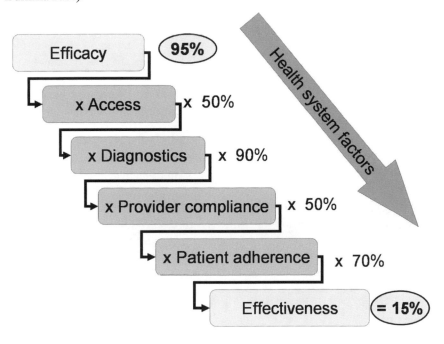

*Figure 41: ACT community effectiveness in young children of rural Burkina Faso*
*Source: Adapted from INDEPTH (2010)*

Untreated falciparum malaria can progress very rapidly into life-threatening severe malaria (Greenwood et al. 2005). A drug against severe malaria should, ideally, be given by controlled rate intravenous infusion until the patient is able to swallow tablets (Warrell 1989). Until very recently, quinine (or alternatively quinidine) has been the treatment of choice for most cases of severe malaria (White 2009). A loading dose of intravenous quinine is usually recommended in order to rapidly achieve therapeutic plasma concentrations. When the patient is able again to tolerate oral treatment, quinine plus clindamycin should be continued for one week or a full course of an ACT should be given (Crawley et al. 2010). Alternatively, quinine can also be given intramuscular or rectal, intramuscular injection being regular practice in peripheral health facilities of SSA. Two large multi-centre trials which compared intravenous artesunate with quinine in adults of South East Asia and in children of SSA have recently demonstrated a significantly higher efficacy of artesunate in the treatment of severe malaria (South East Asian Quinine Artesunate Malaria Trial group 2005, Dondorp et al. 2010). In African children, artesunate was given in a dose of 2.4 mg/kg on admission, at 12 h, at 24 h, and thereafter once daily until oral medication with a full dose of artemether-lumifantrine was possible. This regimen demonstrated a relative mortality reduction of 22.5% compared to quinine (Dondorp et al. 2010). Clearly, quinine now needs to be replaced by artesunate in the treatment of severe malaria, but a Good Manufacturing Process (GMP) formulation of artesunate is still not available (Shanks 2010).

Correct management and supportive treatment in case of severe malaria includes the prevention or early detection and treatment of complications, strict attention to fluid balance, provision of adequate nursing for unconscious patients and avoidance of harmful ancillary treatments (Warrell 1989). Hypotension and shock are often attributable to secondary gram-negative septicaemia requiring appropriate antimicrobial therapy and haemodynamic resuscitation (Warrell 1989, Crawley et al. 2010). Many patients with severe falciparum malaria are hypovolaemic and/or anaemic on admission to hospital and require cautious fluid replacement and/or blood transfusion (figure 42). Young children, pregnant women and patients with severe manifestations, such as hyperparasitemia, are at particular risk of developing hypoglycaemia. As a pragmatic solution, all patients with impaired consciousness should be treated with glucose infusions (Crawley et al. 2010). Various additional adjunctive supportive therapies have been studied over the last decades, but results have been unanimously disappointing (Crawley et al. 2010).

Most cases of severe malaria occur in rural areas with limited access to health services. As such patients can't easily be treated with an oral antimalarial drug, rectal application of an effective drug through parents or community health workers before referral to a health centre may be life-saving. In a randomised placebo-controlled multi-centre trial recently conducted in Africa and Asia, pre-referral artesunate suppositories significantly reduced childhood mortality in patients with a long way to the next clinic (Gomes et al. 2009). Although these results are promising, they need to be confirmed under real life conditions in different countries and cultures (von Seidlein & Deen 2009, Simba et al. 2010).

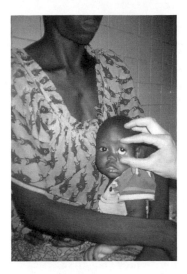

*Figure 42: Child with severe malaria anaemia in rural Burkina Faso*
*Source: Olaf Müller*

### 3.2.2 Home-based management

Most of malaria deaths arc in populations with little access to health services (Greenwood et al. 1987, Snow et al. 1999, Müller et al. 2003). In such areas, home treatment with chloroquine, antipyretics and traditional remedies was until very recently the most frequent response of caretakers to fever episodes in children (Nsimba 1999, McCombie 2002, Müller et al. 2003). However, due to the increasing resistance against the still used older antimalarial drugs in most countries in SSA together with limited access to modern health services, poor quality of such services, low compliance with treatment schemes and poor quality of drugs sold at markets, the community effectiveness of malaria treatment is very low (McCombie et al. 2002, Krause & Sauerborn 2000, Trapé 2001, Müller et al. 2004).

As malaria treatment provided through formal health services is currently not a sufficiently effective strategy for malaria control at least in rural SSA, home- and community-based management strategies are needed to fill this gap. Interventions aiming at improving malaria home treatment by the main caretakers – usually the mothers – can be considered as a complementary strategy. To target mothers through self-help groups has been shown to be a promising approach in the Nouna Health District of Burkina Faso (Kouyaté et al. 2008). Only few studies have been able to determine the impact of complex malaria home treatment interventions at the community level in endemic areas. One study in Ethiopia has measured the effectiveness of treating malaria episodes of young children through their mothers and was able to show a major reduction in all-cause mortality and malaria-specific mortality attributed to the intervention (Kidane & Morrow 2000). In a comparable study in Burkina Faso the intervention was associated with a significant reduction in malaria morbidity, but mortality was not measured (Pagnoni et al. 1997). Results from another study conducted in Burkina Faso supported the efficacy of a home-based treatment strategy on the reduction of severe malaria cases in children (Sirima et al. 2003). However, older studies conducted in Kenya, The Gambia and Zaire using village health workers (VHW) for community malaria treatment were unable to show significant effects of the intervention on morbidity and mortality in young children (Spencer et al. 1987, Greenwood et al. 1988, Greenwood et al. 1990, Delacollette et al. 1996).

Uganda was the first African country which has recently embarked on a national programme of home-based malaria management, which started with chloroquine-sulfadoxine/pyrimethamine and was later changed to ACT (Källander & Nsungwa-Sabiiti 2009). Although this programme demonstrated some success, its application to the increasingly urban populations in SSA is not straight forward (Staedke et al 2009). Finally, it is not clear if home-based treatment strategies would benefit from RDTs used by the respective village volunteers (Lemma et al. 2010). In Burkina Faso, community-based syndromic fever treatment of young children with ACT has become implemented country-wide since 2010, but no data on the feasibility and effectiveness of this intervention are available until now.

### 3.2.3 Intermittent preventive treatment

In recent years, intermittent preventive treatment (IPT) has become an important tool for malaria control, first in pregnant women (IPTp), than in infants (IPTi) and more recently in young children (IPTc) of SSA (Greenwood et al. 2005, White 2005, Greenwood 2006).

In order to reduce malaria-related ill health, regular chemoprophylaxis has been recommended to all pregnant women living in malaria-endemic areas for a long time (WHO 1993a). Most African countries include routine chemoprophylaxis in their official antenatal care programmes. However, in practice coverage of chemoprophylaxis has been limited due to low accessibility and quality of antenatal care (ANC) services as well as problems with compliance (Kaseje et al. 1987, Helitzer-Allen et al. 1993). A survey conducted during the 1990s in four African countries has estimated that less than 20% of women used a prophylactic regimen close to the WHO recommendations (Steketee et al. 1996). At that time, chloroquine was the mainstay for the treatment and prevention of malaria in pregnancy, but the emergence of chloroquine-resistant *P. falciparum* has questioned the efficacy of this well-known drug. Alternative antimalarials considered were mefloquine, proguanil, dapsone-pyrimethamine, and pyrimethamine-sulfadoxine (Menendez 1995, Steketee et al. 1996). Pyrimethamine-sulfadoxine, given in two therapeutic dosages during the second and third trimester of pregnancy, has consistently been demonstrated to be an effective and cost-effective schedule for the prevention of placental malaria and subsequently low birth weight-associated mortality in Malawi (Schultz et al. 1994, Schultz et al. 1996). In a similar study conducted in Kenya, the intermittent application of 1-3 dosages of sulfadoxine-pyrimethamine to primigravid women significantly reduced maternal malaria parasitemia and severe anaemia (Shulman et al. 1999). However, community-effectiveness will depend on coverage and compliance which is not always guaranteed as shown in the population of adolescent mothers in Burkina Faso (Gies 2009). Moreover, it is very likely that the combination of sulfadoxine/pyrimethamine will soon also become a victim of resistance development and not many alternatives exist until today. One promising alternative for this indication is the development of the combination chloroquine-azithromycin (Chico et al 2008).

Intermittent preventive treatment of infants (IPTi) is defined as the administration of a curative antimalarial dose to infants, whether or not they are known to be infected, at specified times to prevent malaria (Greenwood 2007). IPTi can successfully be delivered through the *Extended Programme of Immunization* (EPI) programmes (De Sousa et al. 2010). In Tanzanian children, three doses of sulfadoxine-pyrimethamine given at the time of vaccination with diphtheria-pertussis-tetanus (DPT)2, DPT3 and measles vaccines roughly halved the incidence of clinical malaria and anaemia during the first year of life, and these effects were sustained also in the second year of life (Schellenberg et al. 2001, Schellenberg et al. 2005). In areas of more seasonal malaria as in northern Ghana, IPTi was shown to also provide significant but somewhat lower protection against clinical malaria during the first year of life and no protection during the second year (Chandramohan et al. 2005). A meta-analysis based on the data of six major trials on IPTi with sulfadoxine-pyrimethamine embedded into the EPI schemes confirmed the efficacy of IPTi as a useful tool for malaria control in SSA (Aponte et al. 2009). However, with the development of increasing resistance levels against sulfadoxine/pyrimethamine in many countries of SSA, alternative long-acting drugs are needed for future IPTi programmes. Mefloquine could be an option and further drug regimens are currently under investigation (Gosling et al. 2009). Moreover, combining IPTi with ITNs will likely increase the efficacy of this intervention in SSA (Chandramohon et al. 2005).

Initial studies looking at the effects of IPT with sulfadoxine/pyrimethamine in older children concentrated on the effects on anaemia. More recent studies investigated the effects of IPTc on malaria incidence during the malaria transmission season in West Africa. Two treatments with sulfadoxine/pyrimethamine reduced the annual incidence of malaria by 40% in Mali (Dicko et al. 2004). In Senegal, the application of single dose sulfadoxine/pyrimethamine combined with artesunate on three occasions at monthly intervals during the rainy season resulted in an impressive 87% reduction of malaria cases in children who received IPTc as compared to the placebo arm (Cisse et al. 2006). A large RCT on the effects of IPTc in schoolchildren of Kenya was associated with improved health as well as cognitive performance (Clarke et al. 2008). IPTi and IPTc are less likely to select for drug resistance than chemoprophylaxis, because exposure of parasites to sub-therapeutic drug concentrations is limited, and it is also less likely to impair the development of immunity because exposure to infection will be greater (Greenwood 2006). However, radical clearance of parasitemia may increase the susceptibility to malaria infection and clinical episodes under certain conditions (Ouédraogo et al. 2010).

### 3.2.4 Chemical prophylaxis and mass treatment

Chemoprophylaxis is an important tool for preventing malaria in certain risk groups, such as non-immune immigrant workers, military forces, travellers and pregnant women, and this kind of prevention has also been effective in reducing malaria morbidity and mortality in young children of endemic areas (Warrell 1993, Greenwood et al. 1988, Menon et al. 1990). Chemoprophylaxis is defined as the administration of a drug in such a way that its blood concentration is maintained above the level that inhibits parasite growth, at the preerythrocytic or erythrocytic stage of the parasite's lifecycle, for the duration of the period at risk (Greenwood 2006). However, there has always been concern about the impact of chemoprophylaxis on the development of drug resistance and on the interference with natural immunity in infants and young children in endemic regions (Greenwood 2006). Limited data provide indeed some evidence for significant rebound morbidity in children after stopping chemoprophylaxis, but not for increased mortality (Menendez et al. 1997, Greenwood et al. 2005). Due to such reflections, together with concerns about resistance development and sustainability, chemoprophylaxis for young children has never been implemented on a large scale in malaria-endemic countries (Müller 2000).

Mass drug administration (MDA) describes the administration of a full therapeutic course of an anti-malarial drug to a whole population at risk, whether or not they are known to be infected, usually with the aim of interrupting transmission (Greenwood 2006). A large trial of pre-rainy season MDA with an ACT conducted in The Gambia in the year 1999 was not successful in demonstrating a significant reduction of malaria incidence in the following rainy season, which was attributed to the high transmission intensity in the area and to the insufficient activity of artemisinin drugs against the gametocytes of *P. falciparum* (Von Seidlein et al. 2003). By definition, chemoprophylaxis, IPT and mass drug administration are partly overlapping interventions (Greenwood 2006). Apart from pilot projects at the time of the *Global Malaria Eradication Campaign*, MDA has never become a strategy to combat malaria in SSA.

### 3.2.5 Vaccines

Nature has proven that protective immunity is in principle possible to be achieved but takes time and repeated exposure to the parasites (White 2009). Moreover and already in the 1970s it was shown that both, the passive transfer of immunoglobulin containing malaria antibodies and the active immunisation through administration of irradiated malaria sporozoites were effective in protecting against the disease, but both methods are not really practical (Whitty et al. 2002). Many promising antigens have been identified in recent years and research on vaccine development against falciparum and vivax malaria is ongoing. However, human parasites present a bigger challenge compared to viruses and bacteria, as these are much more complex organisms with multi-stage life cycles in which they express many different antigens of large variability inducing both humoral and cellular immune responses (Hoffman 2004).

There are three principal approaches to a malaria vaccine:

* Development of a pre-erythrocytic stage vaccine
* Development of a blood-stage vaccine
* Development of a transmission-blocking vaccine

With a strong long-term engagement of one major pharmaceutical firm (GlaxoSmithKline, GSK) and support from the largely Gates Foundation-funded *Malaria Vaccine Initiative* (MVI), most work has so far been done in the field of pre-erythrocytic stage vaccine development. RTS,S, an antigen initially developed by the American army which contains the circumsporozoite protein of *P. falciparum* together with a powerful adjuvant, is currently the most advanced approach (Greenwood et al. 2005, Buko Pharma-Kampagne 2010). Initial clinical field studies in The Gambia and in Mozambique pointed to a short-term efficacy of this vaccine of about 30% against clinical disease and about 40% against new infections (Greenwood et al. 2005, Collins & Barnwell 2008). Further phase II trials conducted in Kenya and Tanzania demonstrated a clear association between antibody titers and efficacy as well as the feasibility and safety of applying the vaccine along with other vaccines for children according to the EPI schedule, with a documented short-term efficacy of around 50% against clinical malaria disease (Abdulla et al. 2008b, Bejon et al. 2008). Phase III trials on the RTS,S vaccine are currently under way, but the efficacy of this vaccine under real life conditions and in areas of more intense malaria transmission intensity still needs to be defined (Collins & Barnwell 2008).

Blood-stage vaccines aim at reducing or eliminating merozoites, and quite a number of candidate antigens have been identified, with MSP-1 and AMA being the most advanced in clinical studies (Greenwood et al. 2005). However, naturally existing MSP-1 antibodies were not associated with protection against further falciparum malaria episodes in children of a birth cohort in rural Burkina Faso (Wakilzadeh 2008).

Transmission blocking vaccines are also called altruistic vaccines as all people need to be vaccinated to protect whole communities. The principle is that the vaccination of humans generates antibodies directed at gametocyte or ookinete antigens that can block the development of the parasite within the mosquito (Whitty et al. 2002). Transmission-blocking vaccines against *P. falciparum* and *P. vivax,* considered a key tool on the way to elimination/eradication, are currently in the stage of phase I trials (Greenwood 2005, Targett & Greenwood 2008).

Malaria vaccines clearly are a promising tool for future malaria control, but still need more time for development. In the long-run, successful types of pre-erythrocytic, blood-stage and transmission-blocking vaccines will likely become combined (Whitty et al. 2002, Hoffman 2004).

### 3.2.6 Insecticide-treated mosquito nets

ITNs as a tool in malaria control have gained renewed interest during the 1980s (figure 43). Initial studies were undertaken in experimental huts in Burkina Faso (Brun et al. 1976), followed by a number of efficacy and effectiveness studies with pyrethroid insecticides in different African, Asian and Latin-American countries (Müller 2000). All these studies were able to consistently document significant reductions in the rates of malaria parasitemia and malaria morbidity. Consequently ITNs became employed already during the 1980s on a large-scale in Asia, and this intervention was considered to be more effective and cost-effective than conventional spraying of residual insecticides (Huailu et al. 1995, Bozhao et al. 1998, Verle 1999, Chareonviriyaphap et al. 2000).

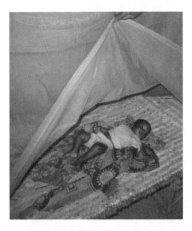

*Figure 43: Child under an ITN in rural Burkina Faso*
*Source: Olaf Müller*

In Africa, a major controlled community trial was carried out in The Gambia (a country with a seasonal malaria transmission pattern and a relatively low malaria transmission intensity of 4-24 infective bites per person per year). In this trial, sleeping under an ITN was associated with a 63% reduction in overall mortality and a 70% reduction in mortality attributed to malaria in young children (Alonso et al. 1991). These impressive results have paved the way for the establishment of a National Impregnated Bednet Program in The Gambia (Müller et al. 1997). An effectiveness evaluation of this program documented an overall 25% reduction in all-cause mortality in children aged 1-9 years, and ITN have also been demonstrated to be effective in reducing malaria morbidity in primigravid women and their offspring (D'Alessandro et al. 1995, D'Alessandro et al. 1996). Results from other trials on the efficacy of ITNs for malaria prevention in pregnancy produced conflicting evidence and were classified as inconclusive by the Cochrane Collaboration (Garner & Gülmezoglu 2001, Lengeler 2004). However, with the publication of the findings from a major ITN trial in a holoendemic area of western Kenya, the use of ITN during pregnancy has been getting more credibility (Ter Kuile et al. 2003).

The results from three further major ITN trials conducted in African regions of very different malaria transmission intensity provided further support for the efficacy of this intervention (figure 44). The first one was carried out on the Kenyan coast (10-30 infective bites per person per year) in a rural population of children under 5 years of age. Protection with ITN was associated with a reduction in all-cause childhood mortality by 33%, and severe malaria cases were reduced by 44% (Nevill et al. 1996). However, ITN had no impact on the incidence of placental malaria, birth weight and perinatal mortality (Shulman et al. 1998). The second large study took place in rural northern Ghana (100-1000 infective bites per person per year). Here, the use of ITN was associated with a 17% reduction in all-cause mortality in children aged 6 months to 4 years, and with additional evidence for a relative protection of neighbours not owning an ITN (Binka et al. 1996, Binka et al. 1998). A third study carried out in rural Burkina Faso (300-500 infective bites per person per year) used impregnated curtains instead of bednets. The reduction in all-cause mortality was 15% over the two years follow-up period, but significant differences were only seen during the first year of the intervention (Habluetzel et al. 1997).

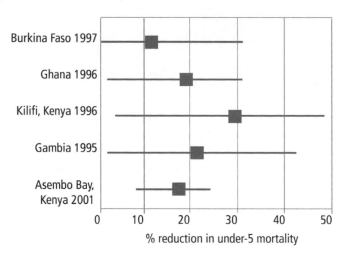

*Figure 44: Under-five mortality reduction attributed to ITN protection in Africa*
*Source: WHO (2005)*

Two meta-analyses estimated the protective efficacy of ITN at around 50% against malaria disease and at 18% against all-cause mortality, with a trend for the protective efficacy to decrease with increasing transmission intensity (Choi et al. 1995, Lengeler 2004). However, as all these ITN trials were only designed to follow children for a short intervention period, possible long-term consequences of young children's protection from malaria through ITN were hotly debated and this discussion contributed to further delays in the implementation of this intervention in Africa (Müller 2000). The major critical question regarding the use of ITN for the protection of young children from malaria concerned a possible shift of morbidity and mortality to older age groups, including a possible increase in the incidence of cerebral malaria. These concerns were triggered by some evidence for overall malaria morbidity and mortality being lower in regions of very high malaria transmission intensity compared to regions of lower and often seasonal transmission intensity (Müller 2000). A possible explanation for such a paradox was the theoretical assumption that under high enough transmission intensity, the age at which functional immunity is acquired may merge with the period of passively transferred immunity. Such an assumption was supported by the provocative findings from a study which compared rates of severe malaria in five epidemiological different settings of Kenya and The Gambia. A total of 5556 severe malaria cases were analysed, and the risk of severe disease was lowest among populations with the highest transmission intensities (Snow et al. 1997). The findings from this ecological study were not supported by further studies addressing this issue. Data from a study in rural Burkina Faso, which was specifically designed to study the underlying hypothesis, provided no evidence for such a risk (Müller et al. 2006). This finding supported the results from extended follow-ups of three large cluster-randomized ITN trials in SSA areas of intense malaria transmission (Binka et al. 2002, Phillips-Howard et al. 2003, Diallo et al. 2004, Lindblade et al. 2004).

First generation ITNs needed to be re-impregnated with insecticide in regular intervals (1-2 times per year), a procedure shown to be not sustainable in SSA (Müller 2000). The development of reliable long-lasting insecticide-treatment, both for the production of long-lasting insecticidal nets (LLIN) (Gonzales et al. 2002, Kröger et al. 2004, Lindblade et al. 2005, Dabiré et al. 2006) and for impregnation or re-impregnation with an insecticide formulation (Yates et al. 2005), has become a technical solution to the problem. However, the longevity of the insecticide treatment also depends on the ITN not being exposed to sunlight, which is not always the case (figure 45).

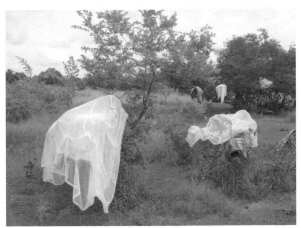

*Figure 45: Drying of ITNs in open sunlight in rural Burkina Faso*
*Source: Olaf Müller*

Today, the large scale application of the ITN intervention in SSA is well accepted in the international scientific community (Whitty et al. 2002, Curtis et al. 2003, Lines et al. 2003, Hawley et al. 2003). A high coverage with ITN would also lead to a mass effect on the mosquito populations similar to what can be achieved through systematic IRS application (Binka et al. 1998, Ilboudo-Sanogo et al. 2001, Maxwell et al. 2002). However, due to major problems with infrastructure, public service organisation, funds and leadership, progress in the implementation of ITN programs in SSA has remained slow until very recently (Victora et al. 2004, Kouyaté et al. 2007). Moreover, a consistent use of ITNs by all household members and irrespective of mosquito nuisance remains a major challenge in all malaria endemic areas, as exemplified by the pattern of use in the Sahel zone during the hot dry season (Frey et al. 2006). Here, people spend the night partly inside and partly outside the house, without moving the ITN around (figure 46).

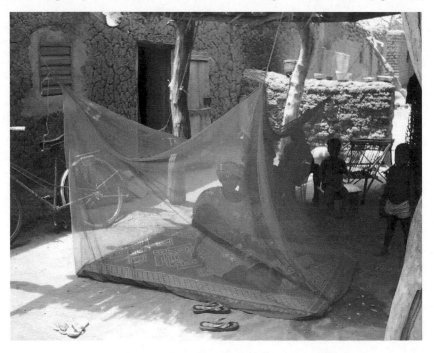

*Figure 46: Mother with her child sleeping under an ITN outside the house during the hot dry season in rural Burkina Faso*
*Source: Courtesy Claudia Frey*

Two approaches for scaling-up ITN coverage in SSA were competing with each other in the international debate. The advocates of the first one considered ITN as a public good and consequently liked to see them provided free of charge (Curtis et al. 2003). The second group has argued in favour of strengthening commercial markets, but has also acknowledged the importance of subsidies for the groups most at risk such as pregnant women and young children (Lines et al. 2003). Those in favour of free ITN distribution supported their argumentation by the evidence from a number of SSA projects and programmes regarding the feasibility of such an approach, the proof of a significant community effect in most areas with high ITN coverage, the reality of a high proportion of SSA populations being unable to pay for such an intervention, and the hope that rich countries would sustain their financial commitment for malaria control in SSA (Curtis et al. 2003). On the other side, those in favour of strengthening commercial markets supported their argumentation by the success of a large ITN social marketing programme in rural Tanzania (Armstrong-Schellenberg et al. 1999, Hansen et al. 2003, Mushi et al. 2003), the important role of market involvement in the success of ITN programmes in Asia, the assumption that free ITN provision would destroy local commercial markets, and the uncertainty of a continuous availability of external funds for ITN programmes (Lines et al. 2003). There was, however, considerable agreement in both groups regarding the need for major donor assistance for whatever approach (Curtis et al. 2003, Lines et al. 2003, Feachem & Sabot 2007). As an alternative strategy, it has been proposed to combine free ITN distribution through antenatal care services with social marketing (Müller & Jahn 2003), and such a model was recently shown to be effective (Müller et al. 2008). Today, free distribution of LLIN to whole communities with the goal of universal coverage has become the standard in most countries of SSA (Gerstl et al. 2010).

### 3.2.7 Indoor residual spraying of insecticides

IRS is the application of long-acting chemical insecticides on the walls and roofs of all houses and domestic animal shelters in a given area, in order to kill the adult vector mosquitoes that land and rest on these surfaces (WHO 2006) (figure 47). The primary effects of IRS towards curtailing malaria transmission are: i) to reduce the life span of vector mosquitoes so that they can no longer transmit malaria parasites from one person to another, and ii) to reduce the density of the vector mosquitoes. Some insecticides also repel mosquitoes and by so doing reduce the number of mosquitoes entering the sprayed room, and thus human-vector contact.

Despite its initial widespread use and contribution to the success of malaria elimination and control efforts, the use of IRS has declined during the last decades (Müller 2000). This was due in part to lack of government commitment and financing to sustain these efforts over the long term, but also to concerns about

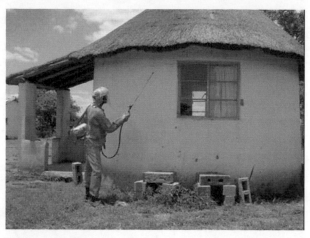

*Figure 47: IRS application in SSA*
*Source: Duffy & Mutabingwa (2005)*

insecticide resistance and community acceptance. However, another important factor has been general disapproval of DDT use due to fears of its harmful effects on the environment and on human health, fears which are considered as unjustified when DDT is used appropriately for IRS (WHO 2006). The main problem was and is that DDT as well as other insecticides are widely used in agriculture and domestic hygiene, leading to massive release of such compounds into the environment. However, despite such considerations and other controversies, DDT is still recommended for malaria vector control in endemic areas (Sadasivaiah et al. 2007).

Numerous studies conducted during the 20th century have shown that IRS has the capacity to substantially reduce infant and childhood mortality in malaria endemic areas (Müller 2000). For example, the malaria incidence was reduced by 90% or more in major areas of tropical Asia and Southern America during the eradication programme through a combination of IRS and other measures (Müller 2000). In Africa, malaria eradication pilot projects demonstrated that malaria was highly responsive to control by IRS with significant reduction of anopheline vector mosquitoes and malaria, although in most cases, transmission could not be interrupted WHO 2006).

In southern Africa, the application of IRS consistently over time in large areas has altered the vector distribution and subsequently the epidemiological pattern of malaria (WHO 2006). The major vector, *An. funestus*, has been eliminated or reduced to negligible levels. The other major vector, *An. gambiae s.s.*, which rests and bites mostly indoors, was also well-controlled. *An. arabiensis*, which does not rest indoors as much as *An. gambiae*, is less affected by IRS, even at high coverage levels, and was responsible for continuous low levels of transmission as well as seasonal increases and outbreaks in this African region (WHO 2006). IRS has clearly been shown to be effective in controlling malaria transmission and in reducing the related burden of morbidity and mortality as long as most premises (> 80% of houses and animal shelters) within targeted communities are treated.

In a single country, several epidemiological patterns and situations are commonly found requiring different interventions or combinations of interventions. These must be taken into account when deciding whether to use IRS. IRS can be effective in almost all settings as long as certain conditions for implementation are met (WHO 2006).

- In unstable, epidemic-prone malaria transmission areas, IRS will prevent seasonal increase in transmission, will prevent and control epidemics and can be used for the elimination of local transmission of malaria.
- In stable-endemic malaria areas with moderately intense but seasonal transmission, IRS can prevent seasonal increase in transmission and reduce levels of infection prevalence as well as morbidity and mortality.
- In stable-hyperendemic areas where very intense seasonal or perennial transmission occurs, IRS, with a higher frequency of application than in the above instances, can reduce the level of transmission and reduce levels of infection prevalence, morbidity and mortality.

There are some situations in which IRS is not a suitable intervention, notably where there are no structures to spray. Therefore, IRS has almost no utility in the control of malaria in forested areas, where personal protection measures are the best option.

There are currently 12 insecticides recommended by WHO for IRS, belonging to four chemical groups (one organochlorine, six pyrethroids, three organophosphates and two carbamates). The choice of insecticide must be informed by the following three considerations (WHO 2006):

- Insecticide susceptibility and vector behaviour;
- Safety for humans and the environment;
- Efficacy and cost-effectiveness.

IRS will only be effective if the target vectors are susceptible to the insecticide in use. The development of resistance to insecticides constitutes a major threat to the chemical control of malaria vectors, as it compromises the insecticide's efficacy. In the past, countries deploying IRS have often been forced to switch to alternative and more expensive insecticides on account of the development of vector resistance (Müller 2000). The potential threat of resistance to public health insecticides appears to be significant, particularly in Africa. Resistance to DDT and pyrethroids in major malaria vectors has been found throughout West and Central Africa, in some areas at a high level, as well as in several parts of Eastern and Southern Africa (Okoye et al. 2008, Ranson et al. 2009). Resistance to carbamates has been found in countries of West Africa, with a mechanism that also induces cross resistance to organophosphates (WHO 2006). The selection of resistance in most malaria vectors is thought to be largely the result of past and present use of insecticides in agriculture (Müller 2000). The precise operational implications of insecticide resistance are not yet fully understood (Takken & Knols 2008).

A comprehensive assessment of resistance at the local level must be carried out before planning any IRS programme, especially in West and Central Africa. The possibility of insecticide resistance calls for the careful monitoring of the susceptibility of malaria vectors to insecticides, and the sound management of resistance (Takken & Knols 2008). There are specific interactions between insecticides and malaria vectors. Some insecticides tend to repel more than to kill vector mosquitoes. Changes in vector behaviour induced by insecticides may have important operational implications, and it is important to be aware of them when selecting insecticides for IRS. DDT is the only insecticide which is used exclusively for public health, and, therefore, unlike with other insecticides, resistance development to it is in theory no longer influenced by other uses such as in agriculture. In the context of resistance management, it is, therefore, advisable to maintain the use of DDT until a suitable alternative is available (Sadasivaiah et al. 2007).

Another major consideration when selecting an insecticide is safety. Insecticides recommended by WHO are deemed safe for public health use under the recommended conditions of use (WHO 2006). Concerns over the safety of DDT, a persistent organic pollutant, have also been comprehensively addressed in the framework of the Stockholm Convention on Persistent Organic Pollutants (POPs). The Convention bans the use of DDT, except for public health purposes. Therefore, DDT can be used for IRS where it is indicated, provided that stringent measures are taken to avoid its misuse and leakage outside public health (Sadasivaiah et al. 2007).

The choice of insecticide has implications for the cost-effectiveness of the IRS intervention. Insecticides suitable for IRS have to be sufficiently stable to maintain biological efficacy on treated surfaces over time, so as to minimize the number of spray cycles needed to cover a malaria transmission season.

DDT has long been the cheapest insecticide and the one with the longest residual efficacy against malaria vectors (6–12 months depending on dosage and substrate) (Sadasivaiah et al. 2007). Other insecticides have relatively shorter residual effect (pyrethroids: 4–6 months; organophosphates and carbamates: 2–6 months). Thus, the use of DDT alternatives might require two to four spray cycles per year instead of one, depending on the length of the transmission season, with important operational and financial implications for spraying programmes.

Currently, the cost of using some of the pyrethroid insecticides is almost equivalent to that of using DDT, but other alternatives might be at least four times more expensive depending on the number of spray cycles required (WHO 2006). The wide-scale use of organophosphates or carbamates in areas of year-round high-level transmission might be very difficult to sustain unless improvements in their formulations result in higher residual efficacy and lower cost.

IRS is a method for community protection, and given its mode of action, the highest possible level of coverage is required to achieve the maximum impact on malaria transmission (WHO 2006). Achieving this level of coverage and timing the spraying correctly (in a short period of time before the onset of the transmission season) are crucial to realize the full potential of IRS. IRS is indicated only in those settings where it can be implemented effectively, which calls for a strong management structure and high and sustained level of political commitment (Sadasivaiah et al. 2007). Transmission control operations based on IRS, or any other vector control intervention, have to be maintained at high coverage levels for extended periods of time, for as long as impact is needed. Operations must be managed by skilled professional staff, based on an analysis of local epidemiological data and a sound understanding of transmission patterns, vector behaviour and insecticide resistance status (Breman et al. 2006).

Also community acceptance of house spraying and cooperation, for example by allowing access and removing some household contents prior to spraying, are critical for the programme to be successful (Breman et al. 2006). Repeated spraying of houses commonly generates fatigue and refusal by householders. Reduced acceptability has been an impediment to effective IRS implementation in various parts of the world (Müller 2000).

### 3.2.8 Other tools and strategies

Environmental modification to reduce breeding sites for the *Anopheles* mosquitoes (e.g. draining, filling, elimination of breeding containers), larval control measures using larvicides such as petroleum oil, different insecticides or the toxins of *Bacillus thueringensis israelensis* (BTI) or *Bacillus sphaericus* (BS), and biological methods based on larvivorous fishes have never been used in SSA on a large scale (Müller 2000, Becker 2003). Large-scale larviciding is probably not very useful in the rural areas of SSA because of difficulties in the location of breeding sites, which are often only of temporary nature, and the need for frequent applications on large surfaces. Larviciding is thus usually restricted to urban areas, refugee camps, and industrial and development projects, and this method is generally not considered to be as effective as IRS or ITNs (Breman et al. 2006). However, under certain conditions BTI/BS methodology is considered a promising additional tool which has been piloted already in some countries of SSA (Fillinger et al. 2003, Fillinger et al. 2009b).

Commercially available mosquito repellents are widely used in malaria endemic areas but mainly restricted to urban populations with some purchasing power. They can be applied to the skin (e.g. DEET) or be burnt inside and outside rooms (e.g. mosquito coils containing pyrethroids). The effectivity and cost-effectivity of these methods is rather low when compared to IRS and ITNs (Breman et al. 2006). Traditional methods to repel mosquitoes in SSA are often based on burning specific plants inside houses (Okrah et al. 2002).

Locally adapted interventions which reduce man-vector contact have recently been demonstrated to be effective in Africa. Simple screening of houses at the windows, doors, and eaves, or over the ceilings, was recently shown in a randomised controlled trial to decrease the number of vector mosquitoes in houses and to reduce anaemia in people living in these houses (Kirby et al. 2009). This is probably not surprising and points to the importance of improving social conditions such as housing to control diseases of poverty (Gimnig & Slusker 2009).

A potential future tool is the development of *Anopheles* mosquitoes containing resistance genes against the malaria parasites (Takken & Knols 2008). Theoretically this is a very nice approach, but it is currently unclear how such resistance genes can be driven into the wild mosquito populations of endemic areas. This is also an ethically challenging research path as it implies large-scale release of genetically modified organisms. Moreover, such mosquitoes may in reality face a selective disadvantage compared to wild-type mosquitoes (Greenwood et al. 2005). Further promising future vector control tools addressing adult mosquitoes and which are under development are entomopathogenic fungi and insect-pathogenic viruses (Takken & Knols 2008)

## 3.3 Cost-effectiveness of malaria interventions

According to a recent statement of 8 internationally renowned economists regarding how to best spend US$50 billion to improve the world in any way, including education, the environment and social services, the three best investments according to cost-benefit analysis were 27 billion US$ for HIV/AIDS, 12 billion US$ for malnutrition, and 13 billion US$ for malaria programmes (Stern & Markel 2004).

A thorough analysis of the cost-effectiveness of commonly used interventions against malaria has been published some time ago (Goodman et al. 1999). The estimated ranges for cost per disability-adjusted life year (DALY) averted were as follows:

- ITNs (nets + insecticide)          19-85 US$
- IRS (two rounds per year)          32-58 US$
- Chemoprophylaxis in children       3-12 US$
- IPTp (pyrimethamine-sulfadoxine)   4-29 US$
- Case management improvement        1-8 US$

Based on new knowledge on the effects of interventions and on their costs for a typical low-income population in a malaria-endemic SSA country, the following estimated ranges for cost per DALY averted were recently published (Breman et al. 2006). In addition, the cost-effectiveness of the recently developed prereferral rectal artesunate treatment intervention is also given (Tozan et al. 2010):

- ITNs (nets + one insecticide treatment per year)    5-21 US$
- ITNs (nets + two insecticide treatments per year)   9-31 US$
- IRS (one round per year)                            5-18 US$
- IRS (two rounds per year)                           11-34 US$
- IPTp (pyrimethamine-sulfadoxine)                    16-35 US$
- Prereferral rectal artesunate                       73-81 US$

All calculations on ITN cost-effectiveness were based on the need for regular re-treatment of nets with insecticides. Given the technical breakthrough with long-lasting ITNs (LLIN), which are now the main product used for malaria prevention in SSA, this intervention is likely to be more cost-effective. IRS calculations were based on four different insecticides, namely DDT, malathion, deltamethrin and lamdacyhalothrin (Breman et al. 2006). One round of spraying is usually needed in areas of seasonal transmission, while two rounds will be necessary in areas of perennial transmission. It has to be considered that the duration of the efficacy of the insecticides used for IRS varies from two to three months with malathion and deltamethrin to six months with DDT (Breman et al. 2006).

These cost-effectiveness estimates were mainly based on existing data on mortality in children under the age of five years and have not taken into account the additional benefits for other household members. All these malaria interventions are considered as cost-effective when using a cut-off value of 150 US$ per DALY averted (Goodman et al. 1999). Cost-effectiveness is also influenced by the level of existing health infrastructure for the delivery of these interventions; the better the health services function the better will be the cost-effectiveness (Breman et al. 2006). Not considering resistance development dynamics, ITNs and

IRS are of about equivalent effectiveness and the choice between these two major vector control interventions is largely based on operational feasibility (Curtis & Mnzava 2000, Müller 2000).

A recent cost-effectiveness analysis of malaria interventions in SSA identified a high coverage with ACT as the most cost-effective course of action and emphasised the importance of considering combinations of interventions during the analysis (Morel et al. 2005). Further developments of the cost-effectiveness of the existing malaria control interventions will largely be influenced by the development of resistance against the insecticides and antimalarial drugs used, and the overall costs for replacing them in case of significant resistance levels.

Little information exists regarding the costs and benefits of converting malaria programmes from a control to an elimination goal. In a recent analysis, the probability that elimination if compared to control would be cost-saving over some 50 years ranged from 0-42%. The authors concluded that financial savings should not be the primary rationale for elimination (Sabot et al. 2010).

## 3.4 Current situation

### 3.4.1 New global health initiatives

Innovation and strengthening of single-disease programmes or other vertically oriented initiatives, which until today are mainly focussed on infectious diseases, has been a dominating feature in recent years in low income countries (WHO Maximizing Positive Synergies Collaborative Group 2009, Sridhar 2010). Such programmes are regularly supported by large Global Health Initiatives (GHI), which documents an increased engagement of private sector, philanthropic trusts, and civil society and GHIs are thus also called global Public-Private-Partnerships. The *Okinawa Infectious Disease Initiative*, which was announced at the G8 Summit in 2000, initiated a strengthened global effort on infectious diseases, particularly HIV/AIDS, malaria and tuberculosis, but also vaccine-preventable diseases and neglected tropical diseases (Reich et al. 2008).

The international frame conditions for malaria control have started to improve already during the 1990s of the last century, after a long period of post-eradication depression during which malaria was accepted as an unavoidable fact of life in tropical regions (Müller 2000). This time the new initiatives clearly focussed on SSA, the continent most affected by malaria. Developments started with a conference of the African Ministers of Health in Dakar/Senegal in the year 1992, and were followed by an increasing number of international initiatives (Müller

2006). Global coordination was taken up by the WHO-hosted RBM partnership, which was founded in 1998 by WHO, UNDP, UNICEF and the World Bank (Müller 2006, Anonymous 2008b). In the year 2000, an important meeting of high-ranking African politicians and representatives of bilateral and multilateral donor organisations took place in Abuja/Nigeria which resulted in the ambitious *Abuja Declaration*. Although this demonstrated the political will to firmly address the malaria issue in SSA, the Abuja goals were too ambitious and the initial funding to low to achieve the targets (Müller 2006, Snow & Marsh 2010).

Low and middle income countries carry the highest burden of disease, but less than 10% of the global spending for health research is used to address the health problems in these countries. This has always been a major problem for malaria control, as the development of new drugs is very expensive and as the pharmaceutical industry has no motivation to invest into the diseases of poverty (Müller 2006). Less than one percent of 1360 new drugs being registered between 1975 and 2000 were targeting tropical diseases (Schirmer et al. 2003). The innovation of *Public-Private Partnerships* (PPP) for drug/product developments (now named *Product Development Partnerships*, PDP) has thus been a major breakthrough. The most relevant PDPs in the field of malaria are the *Medicines for Malaria Venture* (MMV), which was initiated through WHO and the pharmaceutical industry in 1999, and the *Drugs against Neglected Diseases Initiative* (DNDi), initiated through the organisation *Médecins Sans Frontières* (Müller 2006). A number of new antimalarials have now been developed through such PDPs and many more are in the pipeline, particularly through MMV and largely funded by the Gates Foundation. PDPs are potentially beneficial for all partners: products of governmentally funded research are carried on to registration, philanthropic organisations can spend their money useful, and the pharmaceutical industry can improve its image and at the same time invest into markets of the future. The Gates Foundation, with its endowment of 33.5 billion US$ as of the end of 2009, is spending more than 1.5 billion US$ per year for its goals. More than half of these funds go to its *Global Health Programme*, which makes the Gates Foundation one of the major players in the field of international health research funding (McCoy et al. 2009). Besides funding research and implementation activities in the areas of childhood vaccinations, HIV/AIDS, and neglected tropical diseases, malaria is a strong focus of this Gates Foundation programme, having received already more than one billion US$ over time. However, the Gates Foundation has been criticised for exerting too much uncontrolled and technology-driven influence in the field of global health (Müller 2006, Das & Horton 2010).

Already established in 1997 and financed through a consortium of western governments, UN organisations and research institutes, the *Multilateral Initiative on Malaria* (MIM) is another important player in SSA, despite its comparable small budget. Its primary goal is to develop research capacity for malaria in Africa. MIM regularly organises a large malaria conference every few years in different African countries (Müller 2006). The 5th MIM Conference took place in 2009 in Nairobi/Kenya, and was attended by some 2000 delegates (Wakabi 2010).

Today, the most important institution to support control programmes for the three major infectious killer diseases is the Global Fund. It has been initiated through the former secretary of the UN system, Kofi Annan, in the year 2000 and started operating in 2002. The Global Fund has developed a unique lean and effective management structure and is financed mainly through voluntary contributions of the eight major industrialised nations (G8). The three main principles of the Global Fund are country ownership, a focus on results, and strict performance-based funding (Ghebreyesus 2010a). Importantly, a paradigmatic shift towards unrestricted "additionality" of funds was introduced by the Global Fund, which allows circumventing the usual ceilings on the use of general budget support or health sector budget support imposed by the International Monetary Fund (IMF) (Ooms et al. 2008). In the year 2004, the proportion of the Global Fund on spending for control of tuberculosis, malaria and HIV/AIDS in low income countries was already 66%, 45% and 20% respectively (Müller 2006). Of 316 programmes financed through the Global Fund at that time in 128 countries, 61% were in Africa and 31% were malaria control programmes (Müller 2006). In 2008, the Global Fund contributed 57 percent of all international disbursements for malaria control (Global Fund 2010). By the end of 2009, the Global Fund-supported programmes had distributed 104 million ITNs, organised IRS in dwellings more than 19 million times and treated 108 million cases of malaria in accordance with national treatment guidelines (Global Fund 2010).

Another major player in the field of global malaria control financing is the *Presidential Malaria Initiative* (PMI), which was launched by the U.S. Agency for International Development (USAID) in collaboration with the US Centers for Disease Control and Prevention (CDC) in 2005 (PMI 2010). PMI funding has increased from 30 million US$ in the year 2006 to 500 million US$ in 2010. PMI is a large programme focussing on selected African countries, where it supports key intervention strategies recommended by RBM (Loewenberg 2007). By 2008, Angola, Benin, Ethiopia, Ghana, Kenya, Liberia, Madagascar, Malawi, Mali, Rwanda, Senegal, Tanzania, Uganda and Zambia have received funding for their programmes (PMI 2010). However, PMI has been criticised to push for politically motivated programme implementation of low technical quality (Somandjinga et al. 2009).

Malaria control programmes and malaria research also receive contributions through other multilateral organisations (e.g. UNICEF, World Bank), through bilateral agreements with industrialised countries, and through other foundations

116

(e.g. the Clinton Foundation). As none of the existing funding sources for supporting health programmes in low and middle income countries are fully reliable and as there are always unforeseen developments such as the current global financial crisis, there have been calls for more sustainable funding mechanisms such as small mandatory taxes on all global financial transactions or small voluntary contributions on airline ticket purchases, which would overall result in large amounts of funds. This call was reinforced in July 2010 in a presentation of the former US president Bill Clinton at the International AIDS Conference in Vienna/Austria (Clinton 2010).

UNITAID is a newly established international facility for the purchase of drugs against HIV/AIDS, malaria and tuberculosis. It was initiated by Brazil and France in 2006, is now hosted by WHO in Geneva, and has already more than 30 member states and organisations. It is to a great part financed through innovative development financing mechanisms such as a mandatory or voluntary solidarity levy on air line tickets. It has collected more than 700 million US$ since its start, of which nearly half were spent on purchasing ACTs and ITNs for malaria control (UNITAID 2010). Drugs and materials procured are distributed already in more than 90 countries through partner organisations such as the Global Fund, UNICEF, UNAIDS, WHO or NGOs (UNITAID 2010).

The so-called *Robin Hood tax* is a proposed tax (about 0.05%) on all financial transactions, which was launched in February 2010 in the UK by a coalition of different NGOs. This tax can in principle be implemented globally, regionally or unilaterally by individual nations. It could raise up to 400 billion US$ per year, which has been proposed to be used both for development projects in high income as well as in middle and low income countries. The idea has been supported by leading economists, politicians and civil society organisations from around the world. It is conceptually similar to the *Tobin tax*, which was however proposed for foreign currency exchange only. Another difference between the *Robin Hood Tax* and the *Tobin Tax* is that the *Tobin Tax* was intended primarily to stabilise the economic market rather than generate revenue. Controversial discussions around this subject are currently taking place at national, regional and global levels.

The *Affordable Medicines Facility for Malaria* (AMFm) is an innovative financing mechanism designed to expand access to ACTs (Enserink 2008, Adeyi & Atun 2010). It is a new line of business hosted and managed by the Global Fund (Matowe & Adeyi 2010). Financial support for the initiative will come from UNITAID, the UK Department for International Development (DFID), and potentially from other donors. It aims to enable countries to increase the provision of affordable ACTs through the public, private and NGO sectors. In theory, this will improve the access to ACTs and will also reduce the use of artemisinin monotherapy, thereby delaying the onset of resistance to that drug and preserving its effectiveness. To achieve this aim, the Global Fund will reduce the manufacturer sales price of ACTs by negotiating a lower price for ACTs and then paying a large proportion of this directly to manufacturers on behalf of buyers. This should drive the wholesale price down from $4 to $1, and – through 95% donor subsidy the wholesale prices will be lowered to 5 cents. The hope is that retail prices will have a corresponding drop and arrive at an affordable level for poor populations. 225 million US$ have been made available to start a pilot phase of this project in the following countries: Benin, Cambodia, Ghana, Kenya, Madagascar, Niger, Nigeria, Rwanda, Senegal, Tanzania (mainland and Zanzibar) and Uganda. First published results from a pilot project in Uganda have shown a marked increase in the availability of ACTs to young children associated with this intervention (Talisuna et al. 2009).

### 3.4.2 The Millennium Development Goals

The Millennium Development Goals (MDGs), which were announced in the year 2000 by the General Assembly of the UN, are eight international development goals that all 192 United Nations member states and at least 23 international organizations have agreed to achieve by the year 2015. They aim at reducing poverty, improving education, reducing child and maternal mortality rates, fighting infectious diseases such as AIDS, tuberculosis and malaria, ensuring environmental sustainability, and developing a global partnership for development (Sachs 2005). The MDGs contain elements of the WHO constitution as well as elements of the Alma Ata Declaration (see also chapter 3.4.3), but have been criticised of being more selective and less participatory (Müller 2006). Despite such criticism, the MDGs have become widely accepted as a framework to guide international efforts to achieve economic and social development in poor countries (Evans et al. 2005). Below the eight MDGs and their main targets are listed.

Goal 1: Eradicate extreme poverty and hunger

- Halve the proportion of people living on less than $1 a day
- Achieve decent employment for women, men, and young people
- Halve the proportion of people who suffer from hunger

Goal 2: Achieve universal primary education

- By 2015, all children can complete a full course of primary schooling, girls and boys

Goal 3: Promote gender equality and empower women
- Eliminate gender disparity in primary and secondary education preferably by 2005, and at all levels by 2015

Goal 4: Reduce child mortality
- Reduce by two-thirds, between 1990 and 2015, the under-five mortality rate

Goal 5: Improve maternal health
- Reduce by three quarters, between 1990 and 2015, the maternal mortality ratio
- Achieve, by 2015, universal access to reproductive health

Goal 6: Combat HIV/AIDS, malaria, and other diseases
- Have halted by 2015 and begun to reverse the spread of HIV/AIDS
- Achieve, by 2010, universal access to treatment for HIV/AIDS for all those in need
- Have halted by 2015 and begun to reverse the incidence of malaria and other major diseases

Goal 7: Ensure environmental sustainability
- Integrate the principles of sustainable development into country policies and programmes; reverse loss of environmental resources
- Reduce biodiversity loss, achieving, by 2010, a significant reduction in the rate of loss
- Halve, by 2015, the proportion of people without sustainable access to safe drinking water and basic sanitation
- By 2020, to have achieved a significant improvement in the lives of at least 100 million slum-dwellers

Goal 8: Develop a global partnership for development
- Develop further an open, rule-based, predictable, non-discriminatory trading and financial system
- Address the special needs of the Least Developed Countries (LDC)
- Address the special needs of landlocked low and middle income countries and small island developing states
- Deal comprehensively with the debt problems of low and middle income countries through national and international measures in order to make debt sustainable in the long term

- In co-operation with pharmaceutical companies, provide access to affordable, essential drugs in low and middle income countries
- In co-operation with the private sector, make available the benefits of new technologies, especially information and communications

Three of the eight MDGs (4, 5, 6) are directly addressing key causes of mortality in low income countries. As malaria is a disease of poverty, the achievement of all eight MDG would contribute more or less to malaria control and elimination. For measuring progress with MDG 6, which directly addresses malaria, the following malaria indicators were chosen:

1. Prevalence and death rates associated with malaria
2. Proportion of children under 5 sleeping under ITNs
3. Proportion of children under 5 with fever who are treated with appropriate anti-malarial drugs

Whereas indicator 2 and 3 can be measured using national statistics, surveys and specific studies, indicator 1 will be difficult to be determined, as malaria-specific mortality estimates in countries without functioning vital event registration systems depend on instruments such as HDSS-based verbal autopsy (Snow et al. 1999, Müller 2000, Korenromp et al. 2003, Greenwood et al. 2005). However, measuring all-cause mortality developments through national surveys such as *Demographic and Health Surveys* (DHS) will provide already important information for estimates regarding the impact of major malaria control interventions in endemic countries. On the other hand, major reductions in malaria burden may also be accompanied by significant reductions of life-threatening invasive bacterial diseases in children, which will also contribute to achieving the MDG 4 (Snow & Marsh 2010). Finally, the rapid demographic changes occurring in malaria endemic regions have to be taken into account if the MDG shall be reached (Hay et al. 2004).

It has now become obvious, that the MDGs will most likely not be achieved in SSA (Evans et al. 2005, Murray et al. 2007a, Beaglehole & Bonita 2008, Wakabi 2010). Maternal mortality is stagnating, child mortality is not declining fast enough, there are more new HIV infections than the pace of anti-retroviral drug treatment (ART) roll-out, and inequalities are increasing within and across countries. There are many reasons for this, such as not well functioning states, weak health systems, low education levels, lack of donor coordination and insufficient funds (Murray et al. 2007b, Gakidou et al. 2010). As a consequence, there are more and more calls for comprehensive health system strengthening in low- and middle income countries in addition to further strengthening of specific disease control initiatives (e.g. in HIV/AIDS, tuberculosis and malaria). Health systems comprise of four principle components:

- Infrastructure
- Health workforce
- Drugs and other consumables
- Health information system (HIS)

Strengthening health systems and strengthening disease control programmes can be complementary (Ooms et al. 2008, Gyapong et al. 2010, Atun et al. 2010). As a consequence and in addition to traditional funding of health systems through bilateral and multilateral donors, the Global Fund as well as the *Global Alliance for Vaccines and Immunization* (GAVI) Alliance have decided since 2007 to provide additional funding for strengthening health systems (Lee and Harmer 2010, Fryatt et al. 2010). In a joint statement with UNAIDS, the GAVI Alliance, UNICEF, UNDP, World Bank and WHO, the Global Fund has recently confirmed this decision (Ooms et al. 2007). In Rwanda for example, the establishment of a national health insurance scheme was already co-funded by the Global Fund (Kalk et al. 2010).

The *Commission on Macroeconomics and Health* has recently estimated that 38 US$ per person and per year would be needed for a package of 49 essential health interventions in low income countries, but that overall spending on health was only 25 US$ (public and private) per head in 2006 (Working Group 5 of the Commission on Macroeconomics and Health 2002). Public per head expenditure for health in these countries is usually less than 10 US$ per year, with most of this supporting secondary and tertiary care (Ooms et al. 2008, Guyapong et al. 2010). Although development assistance for health has doubled since the adoption of the MDGs, most of this money was used for specific disease control interventions (Shiffman 2008, Sridhar & Batniji 2008). The two working groups of the *High Level Taskforce on Innovative International Financing for Health Systems*, which was created in 2008, have consequently called for more research in the field of health system strengthening including innovative financing mechanisms and harmonised approaches to country-specific support (Fryatt et al. 2010).

### 3.4.3 Revival of Primary Health Care

In September 1978, representatives of 134 member countries of WHO and of 67 NGOs had met in the former Soviet Union and produced the historical *Declaration of Alma Ata* (Müller & Razum 2008). The following 10 chapters of the declaration are nearly as relevant today as they were 30 years ago:

*I*

*The Conference strongly reaffirms that health, which is a state of complete physical, mental and social wellbeing, and not merely the absence of disease or infirmity, is a fundamental human right and that the attainment of the highest possible level of health is a most important world-wide social goal whose realization requires the action of many other social and economic sectors in addition to the health sector.*

*II*

*The existing gross inequality in the health status of the people particularly between developed and developing countries as well as within countries is politically, socially and economically unacceptable and is, therefore, of common concern to all countries.*

*III*

*Economic and social development, based on a New International Economic Order, is of basic importance to the fullest attainment of health for all and to the reduction of the gap between the health status of the developing and developed countries. The promotion and protection of the health of the people is essential to sustained economic and social development and contributes to a better quality of life and to world peace.*

*IV*

*The people have the right and duty to participate individually and collectively in the planning and implementation of their health care.*

*V*

*Governments have a responsibility for the health of their people which can be fulfilled only by the provision of adequate health and social measures. A main social target of governments, international organizations and the whole world community in the coming decades should be the attainment by all peoples of the world by the year 2000 of a level of health that will permit them to lead a socially and economically productive life. Primary health care is the key to attaining this target as part of development in the spirit of social justice.*

*VI*

*Primary health care is essential health care based on practical, scientifically sound and socially acceptable methods and technology made universally accessible to individuals and families in the community through their full participation and at a cost that the community and country can afford to maintain at every stage of their development in the spirit of self-reliance and self-determi nation. It forms an integral part both of the country's health system, of which it is the central function and main focus, and of the overall social and economic development of the community. It is the first level of contact of individuals, the family and community with the national health system bringing health care as close as possible to where people live and work, and constitutes the first element of a continuing health care process.*

*VII*

*Primary health care:*

*1. reflects and evolves from the economic conditions and sociocultural and political characteristics of the country and its communities and is based on the application of the relevant results of social, biomedical and health services research and public health experience;*

*2. addresses the main health problems in the community, providing promotive, preventive, curative and rehabilitative services accordingly;*

*3. includes at least: education concerning prevailing health problems and the methods of preventing and controlling them; promotion of food supply and proper nutrition; an adequate supply of safe water and basic sanitation; maternal and child health care, including family planning; immunization against the major infectious diseases; prevention and control of locally endemic diseases; appropriate treatment of common diseases and injuries; and provision of essential drugs;*

*4. involves, in addition to the health sector, all related sectors and aspects of national and community development, in particular agriculture, animal husbandry, food, industry, education, housing, public works, communications and other sectors; and demands the coordinated efforts of all those sectors;*

*5. requires and promotes maximum community and individual self-reliance and participation in the planning, organization, operation and control of primary health care, making fullest use of local, national and other available resources; and to this end develops through appropriate education the ability of communities to participate;*

*6. should be sustained by integrated, functional and mutually supportive referral systems, leading to the progressive improvement of comprehensive health care for all, and giving priority to those most in need;*

*7. relies, at local and referral levels, on health workers, including physicians, nurses, midwives, auxiliaries and community workers as applicable, as well as traditional practitioners as needed, suitably trained socially and technically to work as a health team and to respond to the expressed health needs of the community.*

## VIII

*All governments should formulate national policies, strategies and plans of action to launch and sustain primary health care as part of a comprehensive national health system and in coordination with other sectors. To this end, it will be necessary to exercise political will, to mobilize the country's resources and to use available external resources rationally.*

## IX

*All countries should cooperate in a spirit of partnership and service to ensure primary health care for all people since the attainment of health by people in any one country directly concerns and benefits every other country. In this context the joint WHO/UNICEF report on primary health care constitutes a solid basis for the further development and operation of primary health care throughout the world.*

## X

*An acceptable level of health for all the people of the world by the year 2000 can be attained through a fuller and better use of the world's resources, a considerable part of which is now spent on armaments and military conflicts. A genuine policy of independence, peace, détente and disarmament could and should release additional resources that could well be devoted to peaceful aims and in particular to the acceleration of social and economic development of which primary health care, as an essential part, should be allotted its proper share. The International Conference on Primary Health Care calls for urgent and effective national and international action to develop and implement primary health care throughout the world and particularly in developing countries in a spirit of technical cooperation and in keeping with a New International Economic Order. It urges governments, WHO and UNICEF, and other international organizations, as well as multilateral and bilateral agencies, nongovernmental organizations, funding agencies, all health workers and the whole world community to support national and international commitment to primary health care and to channel increased technical and financial support to it, particularly in developing countries. The Conference calls on all the aforementioned to collaborate in introducing, developing and maintaining primary health care in accordance with the spirit and content of this Declaration.*

PHC was truly revolutionary at that time as it called for health as a human right and for social justice as important determinants for healthy populations (Lawn et al. 2008). While PHC was not a priority in the high income countries, many low and middle income countries oriented their health system on the PHC concept and thus improved the delivery of health care in their rural areas (Müller & Razum 2008, Rohde et al. 2008). However, in the following years the PHC concept was significantly modified and thus lost its original socio-political focus (Diesfeld 2006). VHWs were rarely sufficiently supported, and the idea of selective PHC which focussed on a few cost-effective interventions took over. An increasing number of vertical disease oriented programmes, which were preferred by the international donors, finally replaced the initial Alma Ata ideas (Diesfeld 2006).

There is a long discussion regarding the benefits and risks of vertical vs. horizontal strategies to improve health in low income countries (Mills 1983, Oliveira-Cruz et al. 2003, Victora et al. 2004, Elzinga 2005). "Horizontal systems" represent the general health services providing prevention and care for prevailing health problems, while "vertical programmes" are designed to address specific health conditions. Vertical programmes are usually associated with poverty and disease epidemics. Such programmes usually have three components (Elzinga 2005):

- Intervention strategy
- Monitoring and evaluation
- Intervention delivery

While the first two components are inherently vertical in nature, the intervention delivery does not necessary requires vertical procedures and may well be integrated in the horizontal system, as it is the case with malaria case management in most of SSA. However, an effective national malaria control programme needs a functioning vertical structure at higher levels such as the regional and national level. Here, sufficient capacity including epidemiological and entomological expert staff needs to be established to make a programme successful (Kouyaté et al. 2007, Newman 2010). Thus, integration of disease-specific activities of the available health force in the periphery (including the private sector), task-shifting if indicated, and a revival of the VHW function are key strategies for effective programmes (Elzinga 2005, Atun 2010). In this regard, the term "diagonal approach" has become established more recently for innovative programme design and financing, which means that large funding for vertical programmes will ultimately increase the money available for the overall health system (Kerber et al. 2007, Ooms et al. 2008, Reich et al. 2008, Atun et al. 2010). However, despite innovative approaches (e.g. "Basket Funding") the coordination and management of the increasing number of disease specific programmes supported by multiple donors constitute a major burden to the weak administrative structures of low income countries (Reich et al. 2008, WHO Maximizing Positive Synergies Collaborative Group 2009). Clearly, a more balanced approach between specific-disease focus and system-based solutions is needed; like weaving a piece of cloth, both the vertical and horizontal threads are needed to form strong fabric (Reich et al. 2008).

In response to the low access to the existing health facilities in rural SSA, the accelerating human resources crisis, and the ambitious MDGs a revival of the PHC movement including the VHW concept is currently taking place 30 years after the Alma Ata Conference (Chen et al. 2004, Narasimhan et al. 2004, Haines et al. 2007, Wibulpolprasert 2008, Anonymous 2008c, Chan 2008, WHO 2009b). As a consequence, VHWs and other volunteers were trained and retrained in recent years in a number of African countries to provide the drugs for home treatment of uncomplicated malaria to households with febrile children (Nsungwa-Sabiiti et al. 2007, Kouyaté et al. 2008, Webster 2009). It is currently under discussion, if even more tasks (e.g. treatment of pneumonia with antibiotics) can be managed by VHW. An additional suggestion is to integrate the roll-out of malaria control interventions with the mass drug administration-based response to neglected tropical diseases (Molyneux et al. 2009, CDI Study Group 2010). All these discussions do also take place in the context of an aggravated human resource crisis in the health sector of low and middle income countries, which calls for innovative management strategies such as task-shifting (Külker et al. 2010). Task-shifting within the health sector has for example been shown to be essential for the current massive roll-out of antiretroviral treatment in SSA (Assefa et al. 2009).

Until today, nearly all of the malaria control programmes in SSA are based on biomedical interventions only (case management and vector control). Very little efforts have been dedicated to behaviour change communication which would clearly benefit from more community participation, one of the key elements of the PHC strategy (Müller & Razum 2008). Knowledge on malaria is often very limited in the affected communities, despite this still being the most prevalent disease in most of rural SSA (Müller 2000, Okrah et al. 2002). Moreover and in contrast to HIV/AIDS control programmes, structural interventions such as women empowerment are usually not seen as specific malaria control strategies. These considerations underscore the need for a multi-disciplinary approach towards comprehensive malaria control and elimination with a strong engagement of social scientists in research and implementation (Williams & Jones 2004, Mwenesi 2005, Stratton et al. 2008).


### 3.4.4 Malaria success stories in Africa

The increasing application of the main RBM tools ITNs, ACTs, and partly also IRS have produced already visible results in some of the malaria endemic countries of SSA (WHO 2009b). However, until now most of the successful African examples are from islands, fringes of endemic areas or smaller countries with significant external support (Müller et al. 2009b, WHO 2009b) (figure 48).

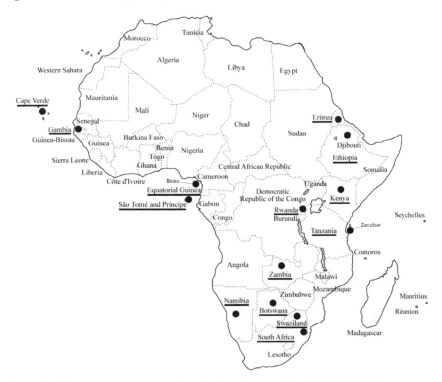

*Figure 48: SSA countries reporting major reductions in malaria burden (2001-2008)*

## Southern Africa

In southern Africa, where malaria is highly seasonal and of low transmission intensity, a number of countries (Botswana, Namibia, South Africa, Swaziland) have demonstrated a decrease in the number of malaria cases and deaths of more than 50% between 2000 and 2008 (WHO 2009b). In South Africa, malaria has only remained endemic in the north-eastern border regions. In the KwaZulu Natal province, the number of malaria cases declined by 99% after the introduction of IRS based on DDT combined with ACT first-line treatment over the period 2000-2002 (Barnes et al. 2005, Sharp et al. 2007) (figure 49). Similar reductions in malaria incidence in Swaziland were probably a result of the intensified malaria control operations in the neighbouring provinces of South Africa (O'Meara et al.

2010). The importance of regional cooperation became very obvious when look-ing at the epidemiology of malaria in South Africa, Swaziland and Mozambique (Sharp et al. 2007). In Zambia, continuous improvements in coverage with ITNs, IRS and ACTs also led to major reductions in malaria prevalence, malaria cases and malaria mortality rates between 2001 and 2008 (WHO 2009b, O'Meara et al. 2010).

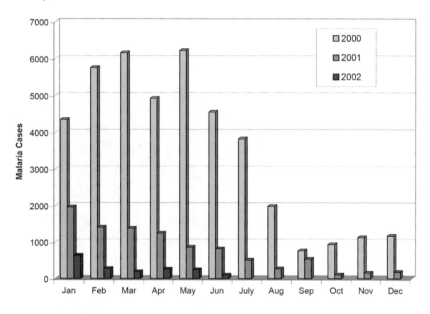

*Figure 49: Malaria cases in KwaZulu Natal (2000-2002)*
*Source: Barnes et al. (2005)*

## The Horn of Africa

On the other side of the continent, a comprehensive malaria control programme based on ITNs, IRS and ACT was accompanied by major reductions in malaria cases and malaria deaths in health facilities of Eritrea between 2000 and 2004 (Nyarango et al. 2006, WHO 2009b) (figure 50). Reports from the neighbouring Ethiopia also demonstrated reductions in malaria morbidity between 2000 and 2007 (Otten et al. 2009). However, the epidemiology of malaria in Eritrea and Ethiopia differs from that of most of SSA as transmission intensity is generally lower and as there is a significant proportion of vivax malaria. Moreover, reduc-tions in malaria burden already occurred before the massive scale up of RBM interventions started (O'Meara et al. 2010).

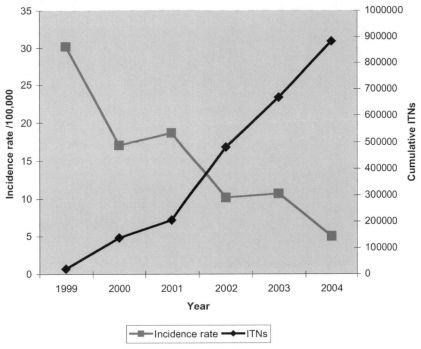

*Figure 50: Effects of control measures on malaria incidence in Eritrea*
*Source: Nyarango et al. (2006)*

*African Islands*

On the islands of Cape Verde, on Sao Tome and Principe, and on Zanzibar/Republic of Tanzania, the malaria burden was much reduced in recent years. The programme in Cape Verde focuses on case detection and treatment, and only two malaria deaths were reported in 2008 (WHO 2009b). In Sao Tome and Principe, high coverage with ITNs, IRS and ACT was accompanied by major reductions in the number of malaria cases and facility-based malaria mortality between 2000 and 2008 (WHO 2009b, Lee et al. 2010). IRS application on Sao Tome resulted in malaria prevalence reductions in young children which were much more pronounced compared to the results of IRS programmes in eastern and southern Africa (O'Meara et al. 2010). In Zanzibar, the comprehensive roll-out of primarily ITNs and ACTs was accompanied by significant reductions in parasite prevalence, malaria cases in health facilities and under five mortality over the period 2003 until 2006 (Bhattarai et al. 2007). The downward trend started already briefly after the introduction of ACT and before ITNs were widely distributed (O'Meara et al. 2010) (figure 51).

Bioko Island belongs to Equatorial Guinea which is a very rich country in the SSA context. Here, a bi-annual IRS programme combined with ACTs, ITNs and IPTp led to significant reductions in malaria prevalence since 2003, but was unable to eliminate malaria (Kleinschmidt et al. 2006, Kleinschmidt et al. 2007, Kleinschmidt et al. 2009).

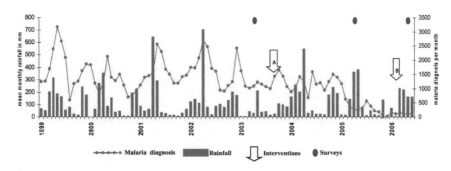

Figure 51: Malaria cases in Zanzibar (1999-2006)
(A=ACT, B=ITN)
Source: Bhattarai et al. (2007).

## West Africa

In The Gambia, surveillance in health facilities demonstrated major reductions in malaria burden over the period 1999-2007, which was mainly attributed to an accelerated ITN distribution. Recent changes in malaria indicators were (Ceesay et al. 2008):

- Major decrease in malaria admissions to hospitals
- Major reduction in proportion of malaria deaths in hospitals
- Major reduction in the proportion of slides positive for malaria
- Major decrease in children needing blood transfusions
- Mean age for malaria admission shifted from 3.9 years to 5.6 years

Apart from these observations in a small and not representative country, existing reports from other mainland West African countries provide not so promising data until today. There are no consistent trends in malaria epidemiology observed in the neighbouring Senegal, and there were even increases in the malaria burden reported from one hospital of Nigeria and from the health facilities of one district of Burkina Faso (Orimadegun et al. 2007, Müller et al. 2009b, O'Meara

130

et al. 2010). The observed increase in clinical malaria cases despite increasing coverage of the population with ITNs in the Nouna Health District of Burkina Faso was attributed to a marked increase in chloroquine resistance during that period (Müller et al. 2009b). Moreover, there were no changes observed in the high prevalence of malaria parasitemia in young children during this period of observation in rural Burkina Faso (Bals & Beiersmann, unpublished).

*East Africa*

In Kenya, a major ITN distribution campaign was associated with a 50% reduction in all-cause mortality between 2004 and 2006 (Fegan et al. 2007). Moreover, there was also the observation of a largely unexplained major decrease in the malaria burden at the Kenyan coast (O'Meara et al. 2008, Snow & Marsh 2010). The malaria parasite prevalence in Kilifi District has declined progressively from 35% to less than 1% since the 1990s, and most of this decline could not be attributed to the increase in ITN and ACT coverage (O'Meara et al. 2010). There are a number of further reports from central Kenya and in particular from the highly endemic western Kenya, which support major reductions in malaria burden in this country in recent years (O'Meara et al. 2010). In the highland country Rwanda, the roll-out of ITNs and ACTs was accompanied by an approximately 50% reduction in malaria cases and deaths in health facilities from 2001 until 2008 (WHO 2009b). Apart from Kenya and Rwanda, the information on the epidemiology of malaria from other countries of East Africa does not look so promising, with conflicting reports from Burundi, Uganda and mainland Tanzania (Mmbando et al. 2010, O'Meara et al. 2010). There is some evidence for increasing malaria burden in the highland areas of East Africa which could be attributed to global warming (O'Meara et al. 2010).

*Central Africa*

There exists not much information from this part of Africa, which is explained by poor infrastructure, continuing armed conflicts, and limited research and implementation capacity, amongst other factors. Available information from countries such as Republic of Congo, Sudan and Cameroon does point to a rather unchanged malaria burden in these large countries (O'Meara et al. 2010).

It thus remains to be seen, whether further progress can be expected in the majority of SSA countries with the ongoing roll-out of effective interventions under the existing scenario of prevailing poverty, weak infrastructure and management capacity, unreliable donor funding, and high malaria transmission intensity, and whether such results are sustainable over time (Anonymous 2009b, Müller et al.

2009b, O'Meara et al. 2010). Measuring progress in malaria control also depends on the availability of quality data which is currently not guaranteed in most of the highly endemic countries of SSA. Data from national health information systems (HIS) are neither representative nor do they provide reliable time-trends, as procedures are changing over time (e.g. increasing availability of malaria diagnostic tests).

Overall, access of SSA populations to effective malaria control interventions remains limited (Snow & Marsh 2010). By 2008, only one quarter of children under the age of five years and pregnant women were protected with ITNs, and the percentage of febrile episodes in young children which were treated with ACT was only 3% in 2006 and remained very low in 2008, despite the international target of 80% coverage for these key RBM interventions (Noor et al. 2009, WHO 2009b, Bhutta et al. 2010).

It becomes more and more accepted in the international health community that a primarily vertical approach to rolling back malaria can't be successful and sustainable without a massive improvement of the general health services in SSA (Müller 2006, RBM 2008). Fortunately this has now in principle also become accepted by WHO and by major funding organisations such as The Global Fund (RBM 2008). The director of WHO, Margaret Chan, has made a clear statement in this regards in her foreword to the 2009 World Malaria Report: *"Ultimately, the power of malaria control interventions must be matched by the capacity to deliver those interventions to all who need them. If we fail to use these unprecedented global health resources to strengthen health systems, then we will have squandered a tremendous opportunity"* (WHO 2009b).


### 3.4.5 The *Global Malaria Action Plan* (GMAP) (2008)

In parallel to an unprecedented political attention devoted to this disease, the global budget for malaria programmes has multiplied in recent years (Greenwood et al. 2008, Mendis et al. 2009). This has mainly been driven by the new international focus on African poverty and the HIV/AIDS pandemic, a better understanding of the humanitarian and economic costs of malaria, and the availability of cost-effective malaria control interventions (Sachs 2010).

By 2009, globally a total of 82 countries were in the phase of malaria control, 11 countries were in transition to malaria elimination, 10 countries were already implementing malaria elimination programmes, and 6 countries were trying to avoid reintroduction of malaria (Mendis et al. 2009) (figure 52). Nearly all countries which are close to elimination are located in the periphery of the global malaria map (Feachem et al. 2010a). The five countries in northern Africa have embarked on a sub-regional malaria elimination programme in 1997; while malaria was eliminated already in Tunisia in 1979, in Egypt in 1998 and in Morocco in 2005, one indigenous malaria case was still reported in Algeria in 2006 (Mendis et al. 2009). None of the countries of SSA are currently in the pre-elimination or elimination programme phase, but a number of countries in southern Africa are planning to embark on elimination (WHO 2009b).

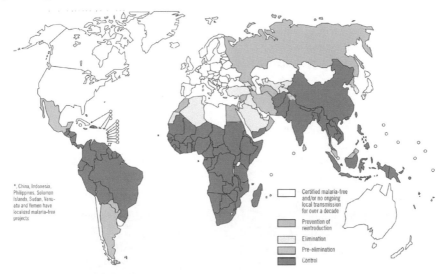

*Figure 52: State of global malaria programmes*
*Source: WHO (2008b)*

The GMAP, which was officially launched in September 2008, is the product of intensive negotiations between representatives of malaria endemic countries and international experts (RBM 2008, Coll-Seck 2008). It aims at a continuous and sustainable reduction of malaria in all endemic areas with the ultimate long-term goal of global eradication. This needs an intensification of control efforts in the holo- and hyperendemic regions and in parallel efforts to interrupt transmission in countries at the margins of endemic zones (Feachem et al. 2010b). Progressive elimination from the endemic margins inward to shrink the malaria map is considered the way forward in SSA (Anonymous 2009b). To achieve this goal, the following objectives have been formulated (RBM 2008):

- Large-scale and sustainable implementation of the available and effective control measures in all endemic countries until the year 2010.
- Reduction of global malaria incidence by 50% in the year 2010 and by 75% in the year 2015 (compared to 2000).

- Reduction of global malaria mortality by 50% in the year 2010 and close to 100% in the year 2015 (compared to 2000).
- Malaria elimination in 8-10 countries until 2015 and afterwards in those countries which are already in the pre-elimination phase.
- In the long-term, global eradication of malaria through successive elimination in all endemic areas.

The amounts of ITNs, insecticides, antimalarials and diagnostic tests needed over the next years to achieve these objectives have been listed in sufficient detail in the GMAP, and also the expected logistical problems during the process of rolling back malaria have been stated (RBM 2008). The costs for the implementation of the GMAP amount to 5,5-7,0 billion US$ per year over the period 2009-2020, which is four times the amount currently spent. Over time it has been considered that the proportion of costs for treatment will go down while the costs for prevention and research will not change much (RBM 2008).

The corresponding *Partnership Work Plan of RBM* for the period 2010-2011 has the following three objectives and accompanying indicators (RBM 2010).

Objective 1: Achieve Universal Coverage

- At least 80% of people at risk from malaria are using locally appropriate vector-control methods such as long-lasting insecticidal nets, indoor residual spraying, and, in some settings, other environmental and biological measures.
- At least 80% of malaria patients are diagnosed and treated with effective anti-malarial
- treatments.
- In areas of high transmission, 100% of pregnant women receive intermittent preventive treatment.
- The global malaria burden is reduced by 50% from 2000 levels, to less than 175 to 250 million cases and 500,000 deaths annually from malaria.

Objective 2: Sustain Universal Coverage

- Universal coverage continues with effective interventions.
- Global and national mortality is near zero for all preventable deaths.
- Global incidence is reduced by 75% from 2000 levels—to less than 85 to 125 million cases per year.
- The malaria-related MDG is achieved: halting and beginning to reverse the incidence of malaria by 2015.
- At least eight to ten countries currently in the elimination stage will have achieved zero incidence of locally transmitted infection.

<u>Objective 3:</u> Prepare for elimination

- Global and national malaria mortality stays near zero for all preventable deaths.
- Universal coverage (which translates to approximately 80% utilization) is maintained for all populations at risk until local field research suggests that coverage can gradually be targeted to high-risk areas and seasons only, without risk of a generalized resurgence.
- Countries currently in the pre-elimination stage will achieve elimination.

# Chapter 4. Challenges for control and elimination

It has become clear already after the failure of the *Global Malaria Eradication Campaign* of the 1950/60s, that sufficient control and eventually elimination of malaria in low-income endemic countries will only be possible if a comprehensive implementation of effective tools goes hand in hand with a massive strengthening of the general health services (Müller 2000, Keusch et al. 2010). This together with the consideration that malaria elimination in the highly endemic countries of SSA will only be possible if new tools (e.g. vaccines or very powerful vector control tools) will become available has now been agreed upon by the majority of malaria experts (Feachem & Sabot 2007, Tanner & de Savigny 2008, Greenwood et al. 2008, Mendis et al. 2009, Snow & Marsh 2010, Griffin et al. 2010, Newman 2010). There is currently no intervention available which would be able to reduce EIRs in these countries below 1, which would be the prerequisite for elimination (Shaukat et al. 2010).

A successive country-by-country elimination of malaria will certainly take place over the next years and decades globally, and partly also on the African continent, but if malaria eradication will finally be possible remains rather uncertain. However, even if a new global approach to elimination and eradication should only achieve a significant shrinking of the malaria map and a major reduction of transmission intensity, morbidity and mortality on the African continent (comparable to what has been achieved some 50 years ago in India), this would already be a very good result (Baker 2008). It has clearly been shown in recent years that a lot can be achieved if the available tools and in particular ACTs and ITNs are made available on a large scale in the endemic countries of Africa.

The *Malaria Elimination Group* (MEG) is comprised of some 40 international experts from a broad range of disciplines. The purpose of the MEG is to make available intellectual and practical guidance, advice and opinions that can be used by countries embarking on, or considering embarking on, a pathway to malaria elimination (MEG 2008). MEG assists countries which are considering or have embarked on elimination (in SSA: Botswana, Namibia, South Africa, Swaziland). MEG held its first meeting in Santa Cruz, California during March 23-26, 2008. The following lessons learned from the history of malaria control and elimination/eradication were summarized during this meeting:

- A single approach for all areas is not applicable.
- Cost-effective surveillance systems must be established and maintained.
- There is need for a clear understanding of the epidemiological situation in each area.
- Population movements (within countries and cross-border) need to be understood and monitored.
- Efforts must include tackling residual *P. vivax* infections, probably through mass-drug administration using 8 aminoquinoline drugs and other available means.
- Technical resources and political focus at high levels must be maintained for long periods (decades in many cases).
- Local/country ownership of programs is a prerequisite which means that responsibility and authority is placed at the national level and should not reside in international circles and/or among funding agencies.
- An iterative process between control activities and research is required – the research and development agenda must be an integral part of any global plan of malaria elimination.
- A systemic approach is required. The integrated application of each control tool needs to be designed within the local health systems context, which also allows i) tailoring operations to local socio-ecological conditions, ii) establishing the partnerships for implementation and sustained financing through a clear definition of roles and responsibilities, and (iii) obtaining social acceptance for all interventions and program activities.

In the next three sub-chapters the major challenges to further progress in malaria control and elimination in SSA will be outlined.

## 4.1 Technical challenges

Beside sufficient funds (see 4.3), the medium- and long-term success of the RBM campaign in SSA largely depends on the efficacy of the existing tools (mainly ACT, ITN, IRS), the development of new tools (e.g. alternative antimalarials, better combination therapies, alternative insecticides, new vector control instruments, effective vaccines), major improvements in the malaria control capacity of affected countries (e.g. training of epidemiologists and entomologists, establishment of quality HIS), and much improved community participation to support the compliance with malaria control and elimination procedures (e.g. engagement of village committees, training of volunteers, improved information/education/communication (IEC) campaigns).

In the field of antimalarials, it remains of major importance to achieve universal access to quality ACT combinations to maximise treatment success and to avoid drug resistance development (Greenwood et al. 2008). This will only be possible, if quality-controlled fixed-dose ACTs will be made available for free or at a low prize through both governmental and private health facilities (e.g. through the AMFm), if routine resistance monitoring is established to guide policymakers when and how to change first-line therapies, if basic and applied research continuously provides alternatives to current antimalarials, and if communities are well informed and supported regarding the correct establishment of malaria control policies. However, engaging with the private sector in the field of malaria treatment may not be without risk. The AMFm for example has been criticised for potentially encouraging antimalarial resistance development and increasing mortality as private health care facilities normally lack supervision and do not use diagnostics to differentiate fevers attributed to malaria from those of other curable causes (Bate & Hess 2009, Kamal-Yanni 2010).

Innovative financing mechanisms need to ensure the continuous access to new antimalarials, as for example shown by the patent-free development of the combination artesunate-amodiaquine through a PDP between the *Drugs for Neglected Diseases Initiative* and *Sanofi-Aventis* (Buko Pharma-Kampagne 2010). A rapid establishment of generic competition has been key for achieving major prize reductions in the field of antiretroviral drug development, and this will be an important mechanism also with regard to access to new antimalarials (Buko Pharma-Kampagne 2010). Global, regional and national mechanisms are needed to address the growing problem of substandard and fake medications in low income countries (Condraun et al. 2008, Siva 2010). Concerning the long-term goal of elimination and eradication, the development of antimalarial regimens containing drugs with a strong effect on *P. falciparum* gametocytes is of overriding importance (Coulbaly et al. 2009, Müller et al. 2009a). It is also likely that *P. vivax* or even *P. ovale* will become more important in regions where *P. falciparum* has successfully been rolled-back, as these parasites are much harder to become eliminated due to their dormant liver stages. As there is currently only one drug with known efficacy against the hypnozoites of *P. vivax* registered, and as this drug (primaquine) is known not to be safe in the large group of patients with G6PD deficiency, the development of alternative drugs which are safe and effective against the hypnozoites will become of overriding importance (Baird 2008, Olliaro & Wells 2009, Wells et al. 2010, Baird 2010). Finally, as every large-scale employment of drugs will lead to resistance development, close monitoring of resistance developments and a strategy of multiple first-line therapies could help reducing drug pressure and thus delay resistance development (Plowe 2009, Smith et al. 2010).

WHO now recommends parasitological diagnosis in all cases of suspected malaria before treatment (Newman 2010). Although the implementation of RDT may well be feasible in the peripheral health centres of rural SSA, it is currently not clear how to deal with diagnostic procedures during first-line therapies provided by VHWs or private pharmacies. Moreover, the diagnostic capacity for other causes of fever will become increasingly important with a successful roll-back of malaria, which again calls for comprehensive strengthening of the overall health system (Newman 2010). Finally, the existence of possibly large numbers of asymptomatic malaria infections with low and sub-microscopic parasite densities will be a major challenge for elimination programmes since such cases will not be detected by standard active and passive case detection methods and may need the introduction of more sensitive polymerase chain reaction (PCR)-based assays (Harris et al. 2010).

In the field of vector control, a better coordination between the agricultural and the health sector is needed to enable insecticides used for public health purposes a maximum lifespan. Routine resistance monitoring has to become established in all endemic countries to inform national malaria control programmes on the most appropriate insecticides to be used. To delay resistance development against pyrethroids, the currently only insecticide approved for ITNs, this class of insecticides should not be used for IRS (Greenwood et al. 2008). Community participation needs to be strengthened to guarantee compliance with ITN use over time (Frey et al. 2006, Müller et al. 2009b). Moreover, simple field tests for measuring of insecticide content on ITNs needs to become established for monitoring of ITN efficacy over time (Müller et al. 1994) (figure 53). Beside increasing support for basic and applied research to develop alternative vector control tools, emphasis should be put on sustaining user-friendly tools which are already available (e.g. ITNs) and on developing resistance management strategies (Kelly-Hope et al. 2008, Takken & Knols 2008). The establishment of the Innovative Vector Control Consortium (IVCC) is thus a step forward (Kelly-Hope et al. 2008). Finally, basic entomological research addressing ecological obstacles to vector control will need increasing attention (Ferguson et al. 2010).

When implementing IRS, it is critical to ensure that adequate regulatory control is in place to prevent unauthorized and un-recommended use of public health pesticides in agriculture, and thus contamination of agricultural products. Pesticide contamination can have serious ramifications for trade and commerce for countries exporting agricultural products (Sadasivaiah et al. 2007). Maximum residual limits (MRLs) of pesticides in food products intended for human or animal consumption are established and strictly enforced by industrialized countries. The standards vary across countries and according to the type of pesticide, resulting in different requirements for exported agricultural products. For example,

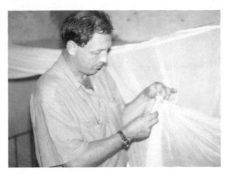

*Figure 53: Measuring pyrethroid insecticide content on ITNs in The Gambia*
*Source: Olaf Müller*

MRL levels for DDT for the European Union usually range from five to ten times lower than equivalent levels for other countries, such as Japan and the United States (Sadasivaiah et al. 2007). Therefore, to export to the European Union, countries must ensure that their products meet much more stringent standards than they must meet for other countries. DDT, as a persistent organic pollutant, is now banned for agricultural use. There is, however, no justification for preventing the use of DDT for IRS based solely on fear of contamination of agricultural products, provided a clear national policy and adequate safeguards for storage, transport and disposal are in place and there is adherence to WHO recommendations (Sadasivaiah et al. 2007).

If true malaria eradication will ever be possible remains uncertain because of the biological nature of the different parasites. It has recently been shown that *P. falciparum* likely originates from gorillas and not from chimpanzees (Liu et al. 2010). Although the main parasites, *P. falciparum* and *P. vivax* currently have no other host than man, *P. malariae* is also found in chimpanzees and the recently discovered *P. knowlesi* is usually infecting primates (Singh et al. 2004). A prerequisite for eradication of an infectious agent is that only humans are affected. In case of zoonoses one would need to also eradicate the animal hosts, which is in most cases impossible (Needham & Canning 2003).

Finally, if control measures do have a significant impact and if they are going to achieve elimination in a number of countries, such developments need to be measured (Greenwood et al. 2008). As malaria becomes controlled in the highly endemic areas of SSA, the pattern of infection and disease will change, with an increasing proportion of older children and adults developing symptomatic disease. However, it is known for long that measuring malaria parameters in endemic countries is notoriously complicated (Korenromp et al. 2003, Greenwood et al. 2005, Hay et at. 2008). There is thus a strong need for improving the HIS

141

of endemic countries and to develop instruments for continuous measurement of malaria parameters through specific surveys, studies and investigations in existing HDSS sites. This needs to go hand in hand with the strengthening of research capacity in Africa (Whitworth et al. 2008, Marsh 2010).

## 4.2 Health system challenges

WHO defines health systems as *"all organizations, people and actions whose primary intent is to promote, restore or maintain health"* (WHO 2000). A health system thus includes not only the governmental health structures but also NGOs, civil society organisations and the private sector. It has been estimated for example that in SSA about half of all health care is provided by faith-based organisations (WHO Maximizing Positive Synergies Collaborative Group 2009). Delivery of health services that are accessible, equitable, safe, and responsive to the needs of the population represents the main output of a health system.

There remain some principle differences in the malaria community regarding the best strategy to achieve comprehensive malaria control, which should be paralleled or followed by local elimination and finally global eradication. While some of the world leading malariologists are still concentrating on biomedical progress and the search for silver bullets, the majority now agrees that only a massive strengthening of the weak health systems in endemic countries will lead to sustainable successes (Feachem & Sabot 2007, Tanner & de Savigny 2008, Greenwood et al. 2008, Lines et al. 2008, Mendis et al. 2009, D'Alessandro 2009, Snow & Marsh 2010). Although vertical approaches to rapid implementation of malaria control interventions promise so-called "quick wins" and may support achieving some of the MDGs in a few countries of SSA, this will certainly not be long-lasting (Feachem & Sabot 2007). Moreover and unlike HIV/AIDS programmes, malaria programmes in SSA do usually not receive the attention they deserve (figure 54). They are placed rather low in the hierarchy of the ministries of health, lack well-trained staff, and do rarely receive sufficient support (Feachem & Sabot 2007). This can be exemplified in Burkina Faso, where malaria is the far leading health problem, but where the national malaria control programme is rather weak (Kouyaté et al. 2007). The current roll out of RBM interventions in this country thus depends to a large degree on the support from external partners such as WHO, UNICEF, and large NGOs (Müller, unpublished observations). However, strengthening malaria control can both contribute to and benefit from strengthening health systems (Newman 2010).

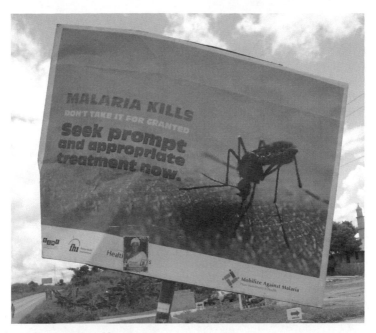

*Figure 54: Malaria poster in Ghana*
*Source: Olaf Müller*

The weak health systems in SSA are facing multiple challenges, such as the "Big Three" (HIV/AIDS, tuberculosis and malaria), neglected childhood diseases (e.g. pneumonia and diarrhoea, various parasite infections), grave maternal health problems, unfinished infectious disease eradication programmes (e.g. poliomyelitis and dracunculiasis), and the emerging epidemics of non-communicable diseases (Beaglehole & Bonita 2008, Samb et al. 2010). This is compounded by the existence of a large number of vertical programmes, which are still preferred by the donors, and by major shortages of health staff. WHO has estimated that, to meet the MDGs, African health services need to train and retain an extra one million health workers until the end of the first decade of this century (Lucas 2005). In governmental health institutions, where expert human resources are in short supply and always in danger of internal and external brain drain, the time needed for coordination and administration of the numerous separate disease control programmes and the many different external donor agencies is lost for programme implementation and supervision. As a consequence, the increasing amount of funds available for malaria interventions can hardly be absorbed by the weak health system structures in most SSA countries (Feachem & Sabot 2007).

The national malaria control programmes clearly need strengthening in the areas of management capacity, supply chain systems, epidemiological and entomological expertise, IEC, and monitoring and evaluation. As the examples from a report of successful large-scale disease control programmes in different countries clearly show, strong leadership, sound management, and adequate and predictable financing were central to the success of such programmes (Feachem & Sabot 2007). The potential large impact sustained quality health services can have in poor populations of SSA has been demonstrated in the Keneba area of rural Gambia, where the establishment of a research unit in 1949 was later accompanied by the provision of 24 hours curative and preventive services through well trained health workers. Under-5 mortality was reduced from 400 per 1000 to less than 20 per 1000 already by 1980, a figure comparable to mortality rates in middle and high income countries (Weaver & Beckerleg 1993).

The malaria community could also learn from the developments in the fight against HIV/AIDS. The HIV/AIDS community was and still is very successful in employing activists to lobby for high political attention and massive financial support (Hanson 2001). With the development of effective drug regimens against this disease in the year 1996, a massive pressure from civil society groups has led to the establishment of comprehensive ART programmes, despite initial scepticism about the feasibility of such schemes in SSA (Müller et al. 1998, Harries et al. 2006, van Damme et al. 2006). This was accompanied by major reductions in ART costs (Gilks et al. 2006). As the current out-roll of ART programmes in Africa is also suffering from the scarcity of human resources in the health sector, HIV/AIDS programmes have integrated ART into the peripheral health services and successfully employed task-shifting within the health workforce (Van Damme et al. 2006, Assefa et al. 2009). It is now hotly debated, if the investments in HIV/AIDS programmes and other more vertically oriented health programmes had more of a strengthening or weakening effect on the global health systems in SSA (WHO Maximizing Positive Synergies Collaborative Group 2009). Whatever the answer will be, it is already clear that the ever increasing HIV/AIDS patient load in SSA can't be managed in a sustainable way without significant strengthening of the health systems of the affected countries (Kober & van Damme 2004, Külker et al. 2010). Africa clearly needs a more balanced investment in human resources, infrastructure, drugs, logistics and other supportive services that will enhance its capacity to deliver health care.

In countries which will move from disease control to disease elimination, a large impact on generalised health services can be expected. The transition from malaria control to elimination demands a major change in strategy: from emphasis on coverage of interventions to emphasis on effective surveillance combined with efforts to prevention of outbreaks and prevention of reintroduction of the disease (Moonen et al. 2010). A reorientation from malaria control to elimination begins with the *pre-elimination programme*, which is considered in areas where the malaria burden has been maximally reduced. A *pre-elimination programme* will usually not start in districts before less than 5% of febrile patients are diagnosed with malaria or before less than 500 malaria cases are detected annually per 100.000 people (Mendis et al. 2009). Most countries made this transition much later, when only a few hundred cases have remained. With the start of the *pre-elimination programme*, all symptomatic cases will receive a parasitological diagnosis and will be treated effectively. At this stage, the programme has to have addressed (Mendis et al. 2009):

- Strengthening the health information system, including entomological surveillance and immediate notification of all malaria cases
- Improving the effective coverage of good-quality curative and preventive health services in all transmission areas. This implies that the whole population, either nationals or foreigners, is easily accessing and using private and/or public health-care facilities, whatever their citizenship or conditions (refugees, displaced, temporary workers, etc.)
- Reorienting public and private health service staff towards the new goals of malaria elimination
- Establishing the national malaria elimination monitoring committee
- Developing the elimination programme
- Setting up the elimination data base
- Setting up a national register of foci (well-defined areas where malaria transmission can occur)
- Strengthening the programme in terms of personnel, resources and logistics
- Establishing a programme of joint activities in international border areas
- Mobilizing domestic funding and necessary assistance from international and bilateral partners
- Advocacy to assure political commitment and continuous funding for remaining transmission foci (especially in the decentralised political and budget context that many countries are experiencing)

The *elimination programme* usually starts when the malaria burden is further reduced to below 100 cases per 100.000 populations per year, where local transmission is limited to clearly defined foci, and where the *pre-elimination programme* has achieved its goals. At this stage, the following programme changes have to be completed (Mendis et al. 2009):

- Training and reorientation of personnel has taken place
- The organisation and physical facilities for the programme have been set up

- Drug policy change to include primaquine treatment for *P. vivax* (radical treatment) and ACT plus 1 day gametocyte treatment for *P. falciparum* has been implemented
- All malaria cases are microscopically confirmed and treated according to national policy, including cases diagnosed and treated in the private sector
- Microscopy quality-assurance systems are fully operational
- All malaria cases are notified, epidemiologically investigated and centrally registered
- Malarious areas are clearly delimited and an inventory of foci has been made
- An elimination database has been set up, including geographic information systems-based data on foci, cases, vectors, parasite isolates and interventions

It is obvious, that such a move from control to elimination will be very demanding to respective health systems. With today's capacity, the health systems of most of the low income countries in SSA would certainly not be able to support elimination programmes (Tatem et al. 2010, Marsh 2010). Moreover, the candidate middle income countries at the margins of the African malaria map need to consider the high costs of such a move. In such countries, malaria interventions will clearly be prioritized and possibly delivered at the expense of other essential health services (Shah 2010).

## 4.3 Financial challenges

Between 2001 and 2006, official annual overseas development assistance for health (DAH) has increased from 5.6 billion US$ to 13.8 billion US$ (WHO Maximizing Positive Synergies Collaborative Group 2009). In addition, non-official DAH has also increased substantially due to the emergence of numerous large GHIs (e.g. Global Fund, GAVI, US Presidential Initiatives on HIV/AIDS and malaria, specific programmes of the World Bank, Gates Foundation, NGOs) (WHO Maximizing Positive Synergies Collaborative Group 2009, Sachs 2010). In 2007, the new GHIs provided 67% of all external funding for HIV/AIDS, 57% for tuberculosis, and 60% for malaria programmes (WHO Maximizing Positive Synergies Collaborative Group 2009). Despite such promising increases in health funding, low-income countries still have to find almost 75% of their health funding in domestic sources (Evans & Etienne 2010) and out-of-pocket payments are still the main source for financing health care; out-of-pocket spending has been estimated to account for 60% of total health spending in low income countries as compared to 20% in high income countries (WHO Maximizing Positive Synergies Collaborative Group 2009). Overall public financing of health through domestic sources also increased substantially in recent years in low and middle income countries, but decreased in many low income countries of SSA. While conditional dept relief had no effect, DAH had a significantly negative effect on domestic governmental spending on health in SSA countries, which is cause for concern (Lu et al. 2010). In 2009, only three African countries met the target of spending 15% of their budgets on health (Wakabi 2010). The average budget allocation to health in Africa is 9% compared to 15% and 17% in Europe and the USA, and most countries spend less than half of the WHO recommended minimum package of 40 US$ per person on health (Wakabi 2010).

The RBM partnership has grown exponentially since its start in 1998 to become a strong coalition of more than 500 partners (Anonymous 2008). Donor funding for malaria control has increased dramatically from only 18 million US$ in 1998 to 1.5 billion US$ in the year 2007; in SSA, 82% of the budgets for malaria control now comes from external donors (RBM 2008, Anonymous 2009). The Global Fund round 7 and 8 had approved a total of 1 and 3 billion US$ respectively for malaria control, and the PMI and the World Bank (WB) Booster Programme have promised further large funds for malaria control (Anonymous 2009, Ghebreyesus 2010b). By the end of 2009, the Global Fund had approved 5.3 billion US$ for 191 malaria grants in 82 countries (Snow & Marsh 2010). New pledges of donors will enable programmes already approved to continue at least until 2013 (Watson 2010, Kazatchkine 2010). All this is good news. However, average annual funding for malaria per head was still below 1 US$ in most of the endemic countries of SSA by 2007 (Teklehaimanot et al. 2007, Snow et al. 2008) and to achieve the ambitious goals of the *Global Malaria Action Plan*, at least 62 billion US$ are needed by 2020 (Anonymous 2008) (table 7). It may also be asked if this is realistic and justified given the multiple competing health problems in endemic countries, the global financial crisis, and the likely long-term donor fatigue after aggressive short-term goals will have been achieved (Feachem & Sabot 2008, Feachem & Phillips 2009, Mendis et al. 2009, Snow & Marsh 2010).

| Cost (US$ millions) | 2009 | 2010 | 2015 | 2020 | 2025 |
|---|---|---|---|---|---|
| Prevention cost | 3,728 | 3,982 | 3,724 | 3,864 | 2,576 |
| Case management cost | 968 | 1,359 | 550 | 226 | 87 |
| Program cost | 638 | 839 | 764 | 787 | 714 |
| *Global control and elimination cost* | *5,335* | *6,180* | *5,037* | *4,877* | *3,378* |
| *Research and development cost* | *759* | *759* | *800* | *681* | *460* |
| Total cost | 6,094 | 6,939 | 5,837 | 5,559 | 3,838 |

*Table 7: Estimated costs of the Global Malaria Action Plan of RBM*
*Source: RBM (2008)*

The idea to turn the Global Fund and the GAVI Alliance into a "Global Health Fund", a "Global Fund for the health MDGs" or a "World Health Insurance" has recently been introduced to the international discussion (Ooms et al. 2008, Cornetto et al. 2009, Anonymous 2010). Such a fund could aim to support public health expenditure of 40 US$ per person per year in 54 low-income countries and this would need about 28 billion US$ per year (Ooms et al. 2008). The conservative estimate of 40 US$ (taking into consideration domestic resource mobilisation for public health in the order of 15US$ per person per year) was calculated to cover a set of priority interventions with the infrastructure necessary to deliver them, but not the costs of training new personnel, preventive programmes, emergency care or referral hospitals (Ooms et al. 2008, Sachs 2010). The sum of 28 billion US$ seems impressive but appears rather modest if compared to the 300 billion US$ spent globally in agricultural subsidies, the 1.5 trillion US$ spent for military expenditures, and the total of 6 trillion spent for global health every year (Garrett et al. 2009, Gostin 2010).

The combined gross domestic product (GDP) of the Organisation of Economic Co-operation and Development (OECD) member countries was estimated at 36 trillion US$ in 2006. If 0.7% of the GDP of OECD countries would be delivered for foreign assistance as promised already in 1970, and if 15% of that were allocated for health sector support, 38 billion US$ per year would be available (Ooms et al. 2008, Gostin 2010). A Global Health Fund thus appears to be feasible but would need several times the annual funding level of the Global Fund to arrive at the required 28 billion US$ per year. In analogy to the AIDS activism and "right to health" approach-triggered exemption of HIV/AIDS programmes and other vertical GHIs from the IMF-driven paradigm of national financial autonomy, a Global Health Fund also needs to abolish the idea that countries receiving external assistance will soon be able to finance their health services through domestic sources (Cornetto et al. 2009). Such a Fund would be a major step forward to the long-needed harmonisation of global health financing and would enable a sustainable delivery of comprehensive prevention and treatment services for specific diseases through improved general health services (Cornetto et al. 2009). Some 60 years after the Universal Declaration of Human Rights and some 30 years after the Alma-Ata Declaration on PHC, a sufficiently equipped and correctly administered Global Health Fund would also support the ongoing process of putting the *Right to Health* into practice (Pillay 2008).

# Conclusions

More than half a century ago, the global community embarked on an ambitious malaria eradication campaign. By definition this campaign was a failure, although it finally eliminated malaria in all of the high income countries and reduced the burden of this disease significantly in endemic areas of low and middle income countries, with the exception of the largely neglected African continent. Beside technical aspects such as resistance development of vector mosquitoes to insecticides and malaria parasites to antimalarial drugs, the main reason for the failure of the campaign to achieve its goal was the weak health systems in poor tropical countries.

In Africa, malaria control was largely limited to syndromic fever treatment with chloroquine for the last decades. The emergence of wide-spread *P. falciparum* resistance to chloroquine during the 1990s with its large impact on child mortality was a wake-up call for the international community. Most of the global malaria burden nowadays is in SSA and this is amongst the major impediments for economic development on this continent beside HIV/AIDS. With the event of the MDGs, Africa has received much renewed attention since the year 2000. An ever increasing number of new GHIs is now trying to address most of the health problems in SSA, including the release of large funds for malaria control. This has also triggered a renewed discussion about global malaria eradication. In analogy to the time of the first malaria eradication campaign, there are now two new and powerful tools available: synthetic pyrethroids for vector control and artemisinin derivates for antimalarial combination therapy. Despite well documented effectiveness in country-wide applications of these tools, it appears rather unlikely to achieve malaria elimination in the highly malaria endemic areas of SSA without further tools (e.g. vaccines) becoming available. However, the major barrier to successful disease control including malaria control programmes is the weak health systems in the majority of SSA countries. It is thus reassuring that most of the donors and representatives of new GHIs are now considering to provide funds for improving health services in addition to funding of specific disease programmes.

The development of a Global Health Fund with sufficient and sustainable amounts of money provided by the high income countries could be the way forward. Such a Fund would concentrate on supporting PHC in all low-income countries including integration of the activities of the various vertically oriented GHIs.

If this would receive the political and financial support it deserves, this would be a major step forward for achieving the MDGs. Beside a true commitment of the international community to a long-term response, renewed global efforts on strengthening health systems would need to be backed up by a strong, well-funded, and politically supported WHO.

Today, it appears to be possible to eliminate malaria from selected countries in southern Africa and to achieve major reductions in the disease burden in the rest of SSA, but wide-spread elimination will only take place if overall development leads to better educated populations, much reduced poverty, and well functioning health systems with a clear focus on PHC.

# Acknowledgments

I like to thank all my colleagues from the *Institute of Public Health* at the Heidelberg University and from the *Centre de Recherche en Santé de Nouna*, who have greatly supported me over the last couple of years in my research activities on malaria in Africa and beyond. I am also indebted to Brian Greenwood, who provided me with fundamental guidance and in depth advice over the last 15 years on this topic. Moreover, I like to acknowledge the financial support I have received from the German Science Foundation in the frame of the special research programme "Control of tropical infectious diseases" (SFB 544) and the professional support from my Heidelberg colleagues during the 12 years of joint research activities in Heidelberg/Germany.

Special thanks go to my colleagues Yesim Tozan, Albrecht Jahn and Frank Mockenhaupt for their critical reading, constructive comments and helpful corrections on the manuscript, and to the editor of this book series, Oliver Razum. I am also grateful to the members of my working group for various supports during the production of the final manuscript, in particularly to Valérie Louis, Claudia Beiersmann, Nobila Ouédraogo and Farida Kamrudin. Finally I like to thank my wife, Christina, and my children, Milena and Maximilian, for their great patience during the long evening and weekend hours I have spent working on the finalisation of this book.

This book is dedicated to the children of SSA, who have the right of access to functioning health services and who deserve a malaria-free future.

# References

Abacassamo F, Enosse S, Aponte JJ, Gómez-Olivé FX, Quintó L, Mabunda S, Barreto A, Magnussen P, Ronn AM, Thompson R, Alonso PL. Efficacy of chloroquine, amodiaquine, suphadoxine-pyrimethamine and combination therapy with artesunate in Mosambican children with non-complicated malaria. *Tropical Medicine & International Health* 9: 200–208 (2004)

Abdulla S, Sagara I, Borrmann S, D'Alessandro U, González R, Hamel M, Ogutu B, Mårtensson A, Lyimo J, Maiga H, Sasi P, Nahum A, Bassat Q, Juma E, Otieno L, Björkman A, Beck HP, Andriano K, Cousin M, Lefèvre G, Ubben D, Premji ZK. Efficacy and safety of artemether-lumefantrine dispersible tablets compared with crushed commercial tablets in African infants and children with uncomplicated malaria: a randomised, single-blind, multicentre. *The Lancet* 372: 1819–27 (2008a)

Abdulla S, Oberholzer R, Juma O, Kubhoja S, Machera F, Membi C, Omari S, Urassa A, Mshinda H, Jumanne A, Salim N, Shomari M, Aebi T, Schellenberg DM, Carter T, Villafana T, Demoitié M, Dubois M, Leach A, Lievens M, Vekemans J, Cohen J, Ballou WR, Tanner M. Safety and Immunogenicity of RTS,S/AS02D Malaria Vaccine in Infants. *The New England Journal of Medicine* 359: 2533–44 (2008b)

Abu-Raddad LJ, Patnaik P, Kublin JG. Dual infection with HIV and malaria fuels the spread of both diseases in sub-Saharan Africa. *Science* 314: 1603–1606 (2006)

Adeyi O, Atun R. Viepoint: Universal access to malaria medicines: innovation in financing and delivery. *The Lancet* 376: 1869–71 (2010)

Agyepong IA. Malaria: Ethnomedical perception and practice in an Adangbe farming community and implications for control. *Social Science and Medicine* 35: 131–137 (1992)

Ahorlu CK, Dunyo SK, Afari EA, Koram KA, Nkrumah FK. Malaria-related beliefs and behaviour in southern Ghana: implications for treatment, prevention and control. *Tropical Medicine & International Health* 2:488–99 (1997)

Aikins MK, Pickering H, Alonso L, D'Alessandro U, Lindsay W, Todd J, Greenwood BM. A malaria control trial using insecticide-treated bed nets and targeted chemoprophlaxis in a rural area of The Gambia, West Africa. *Transactions of the Royal Society of Tropical Medicine and Hygiene* 87 (supplement 2): 25–30 (1993)

Alonso P, Lindsay S, Armstrong J, Conteh M, Hill A, David P, Fegan G, De Francisco A, Hall A, Shenton F, Cham K, Greenwood B. The effect of insecticide-treated bednets on mortality in Gambian children. *The Lancet* 337: 1499–1502 (1991)

Anonymous. Editorial – Malaria Control and Primary Health Care. *The Lancet* 322: 963–964 (1983)

Anonymous. Kwa Zulo Natal's successful fight against malaria. *PLoS Medicine* 2: e371 (2005)

Anonymous. Nobel award opens old wounds. *The Lancet Infectious Diseases* 8: 659 (2008a)

Anonymous. Rolling back malaria – the next 10 years. *The Lancet* 372: 1193 (2008b)

Anonymous. Editorial: Margaret Chan puts primary health care centre stage at WHO. *The Lancet* 371: 1811 (2008c)

Anonymous. Resistance to the Affordable Medicines Facility for malaria? *The Lancet* 373: 1400 (2009a)

Anonymous. Maintaining momentum for malaria elimination. *The Lancet* 347: 266 (2009b)

Anonymous. Another step towards preventing artemisinin resistance. *The Lancet* 375: 956 (2010a)

Anonymous. The Global Fund: replenishment and redefinition in 2010. *The Lancet* 375: 865 (2010b)

Ansah EK, Narh-Bana S, Epokor M, Akanpigbiam S, Quartey AA, Gyanpong J, Whitty CJM. Rapid testing for malaria in settings where microscopy is available and peripheral clinics where only presumptive treatment is available: a randomised controlled trial in Ghana. *BMJ* 340: c930 (2010)

Anstey NM, Russell B, Yeo TW, Price RN. The pathophysiology of vivax malaria. *Trends in Parasitology* 25: 220–27 (2009)

Aponte JJ, Schellenberg D Egan A, Breckenridge A, Carneiro I, Critchley J, Danquah I, Dodoo A, Kobbe R, Lell B, May J, Premji Z, Sanz S, Sevene E, Soulaymani-Becheikh R, Winstanley P, Adjei S, Anemana S, Chandramohan D, Issifou S, Mockenhaupt F, Owusu-Agyei S, Greenwood B, Grobusch MP, Kremsner PG, Macete E, Mshinda H, Newman RD, Slutsker L, Tanner M, Alonso P, Menendez C. Efficacy and safety of intermittent preventive treatment with sulfadoxine-pyrimethamine for malaria in African infants: a pooled analysis of six randomised, placebo-controlled trials. *The Lancet* 374:1533–42 (2009)

Armstrong-Schellenberg J, Abdulla S, Minja H. KINET: a social marketing programme of treated nets and net treatment for malaria control in Tanzania, with evaluation of child health and long-term survival. *Transactions of the Royal Society of Tropical Medicine and Hygiene* 93: 225–31 (1999)

Assefa Y, Jerene D, Lulseged S, Ooms G, Damme WV. Rapid Scale-Up of Antiretroviral Treatment in Ethiopia: Successes and System-Wide Effects. *PloS Medicine* 6,4,e1000056 (2009)

Atun R, Weil DEC, Eang MT, Mwakyusa D. Health-system strenghening and tuberculosis control. *The Lancet* 375: 2169–78 (2010)

Baird JK. Real-World Therapies and the Problem of Vivax Malaria. *New England Journal of Medicine* 359: 2601–03 (2008)

Baird JK. Eliminating malaria – all of them. *The Lancet* 376: Early online publication, 29 October (2010)

Baker TD. Malaria eradication in India: a failure? *Science* 319: 1616 (2008)

Barnes KI, Durrheim DN, Little F, Jackson A, Mehta U, Allen E, Dlamini SS, Tsoka J, Bredenkamp B, Mthembu DJ, Nicholas J, White NJ, Brian L. Sharp BL. Effect of Artemether-Lumefantrine Policy and Improved Vector Control on Malaria Burden in KwaZulu–Natal, South Africa. *PLoS Medicine* 2: e330 (2005)

Basco LK. Molecular epidemiology of malaria in Cameroon. XIX. Quality of antimalarial drugs used for self-medication. *American Journal of Tropical Medicine and Hygiene* 70: 245–50 (2004)

Bate R, Hess K. Affordable Medicines Facility for malaria. *The Lancet* 9: 396–7 (2009)

Baume C, Helitzer D, Kachur SP. Patterns of care for childhood malaria in Zambia. *Social Science and Medicine* 51, 1491–1503 (2000)

Beaglehole R, Bonita R. Global Public Health: a scorecard. *The Lancet* 372: 1988–96 (2008)

Becher H, Kynast-Wolf G, Sié A, Ndugwa R, Ramroth H, Kouyaté B, Müller O. Patterns of malaria, cause-specific and all cause mortality in a malaria endemic area of West Africa. *American Journal of Tropical Medicine and Hygiene* 78: 106–113 (2008)

Becker N. Mosquitoes and their control. Springer, ISBN 978-0-306-47360-9 (2003)

Beiersmann C, Sanou A, Wladarsch E, De Allegri M, Kouyaté B, Müller O. Malaria in rural Burkina Faso: local illness concepts, patterns of traditional treatment and influence on health-seeking behaviour. *Malaria Journal* 6: 106 (2007)

Bejon P, Lusingu J, Olotu A, Leach A, Lievens M, Vekemans J, Mshamu S, Lang T, Gould J, Dubois M, Demoitié M, Jan-Francois Stallaert J, Vansadia P, Carter T, Njuguna P, Ken O, Malabeja AA, Abdul O, Gesase S, Mturi N, Drakeley CJ, Savarese B, Villafana T, Ballou WR, Cohen J, Riley EM, Lemnge MM, Marsh K, Seidlein L. Efficacy of RTS,S/AS01E Vaccine against Malaria in Children 5 to 17 Months of Age. *The New England Journal of Medicine* 359: 2521–32 (2008)

Berkley JA, Lowe BS, Mwangi I, Williams T, Bauni E, Mwarumba S, Ngetsa C, Slack MPE, Njenga S, Hart A, Maitland K, English M, Marsh K, Scott JAG. Bacteremia among Children Admitted to a Rural Hospital in Kenya. *The New England Journal of Medicine* 352:39–47 (2005)

Berkley JA, Mwarumba S, Bramham K, Lowe B, Marsh K. Bacteriaemia complicating severe malaria in children. *Transactions of the Royal Society of Tropical Medicine and Hygiene* 93:283–86 (1999)

Bhattarai A, Ali AS, Kachur SP, Mårtensson A, Abbas AK, Khatib R, Al-Mafazy AW, Ramsan M, Rotllant G, Gerstenmaier JF, Molteni F, Abdulla S, Montgomery SM, Kaneko A, Björkman A. Impact of artemisinin-based combination therapy and insecticide-treated nets on malaria burden in Zanzibar. *PLoS Medicine* 4: e309 (2007)

Bhutta ZA, Chopra M, Axelson H, Berman P, Boerma T, Bryce J, Bustreo F, Cavagnero E, Cometto G, Daelmans B, de Francisco A, Fogstad H, Gupta N, Laski L, Lawn J, Maliqi B, Mason E, Pitt C, Requejo J, Starrs A, Victora CG, Wardlaw T. Countdown to 2015 decade report (2000–10): taking stock of maternal, newborn, and child survival. *The Lancet* 375: 2032–44 (2010)

Binka F, Kubaje A, Adjuik M, Williams L, Lengeler C, Maude G, Armah G, Kajihara B, Adiamah J, Smith P.: Impact of permethrin impregnated bednets on child mortality in Kassena-Nankana district, Ghana: a randomized controlled trial. *Tropical Medicine & Interntional Health* 1: 147–54 (1996)

Binka F, Indome F, Smith T. Impact of spacial distribution of permethrin-impregnated bednets on child mortality in rural northern Ghana. *American Journal of Tropical Medicine and Hygiene* 59: 80–85 (1998)

Binka FN, Hodgson A, Adjuik M, Smith T. Mortality in a seven-and-a-half-year follow-up of a trial of insecticide-treated mosquito nets in Ghana. *Transactions of the Royal Society of Tropical Medicine and Hygiene* 96: 597–99 (2002)

Bisoffi Z, Sirima BS, Angheben A, Lodesani C, Gobbi F, Tinto H, Van den Ende J. Rapid malaria diagnostic tests vs. Clinical management of malaria in rural Burkina Faso: safety and effect on clinical decisions. A randomized trial. *Tropical Medicine & International Health* 14: 491–98 (2009)

Björkman A, Martinsson A. Risks and benefits of targeted malaria treatment based on rapid diagnostic test results. *Clinical Infectious Diseases* 51: 512–14 (2010)

Black RE, Cousens S, Johnson HL, Lawn JE, Rudan I, Bassani DG, Jha P, Campbell H, Walker CF, Cibulskis R, Eisele T, Liu L, Mathers C. Global, regional, and national causes of child mortality in 2008: a systematic analysis. *The Lancet* 375: 1969–87 (2010)

Bloland P, Lackritz E, Kazembe P, Were J, Steketee R, Campbell C. Beyond chloroquine: implications of drug resistance for evaluating malaria therapy efficacy and treatment policy in Africa. *Journal of Investigative Dermatology* 167: 932–937 (1993)

Bloland P, Slutsker L, Steketee W, Wirima J, Heymann D, Breman J. Rates and risk factors for mortality during the first two years of life in rural Malawi. *American Journal of Tropical Medicine and Hygiene* 55 (supplement): 82–86 (1996)

Bloland P, Kazembe P, Watkins W, Doumbo O, Nwanyanwu O, Ruebush T. Malarone-donation programme in Africa. *The Lancet* 350: 1624–1625 (1997)

Bouvier P, Breslow N, Doumbo O, Robert C, Picquet M, Mauris A, Dolo A, Dembele H, Delley V, Rougement A. Seasonality, malaria, and impact of prophylaxis in a West African village. II. Effect on birthweight. *American Journal of Tropical Medicine and Hygiene* 56: 384–389 (1997a)

Bouvier P, Doumbo O, Breslow N, Robert C, Mauris A, Picquet M, Kouriba B, Dembele H, Delley V, Rougement A. Seasonality, malaria, and impact of prophylaxis in a West African village. I. Effect on anaemia in pregnancy. *American Journal of Tropical Medicine and Hygiene* 56: 378–383 (1997b)

Bozhao X, Xianqi X, Webber R, Lines J. Comparison of the effect of insecticide-treated bednets and DDT residual spraying on the prevalence of malaria transmitted by *An. anthropophagus* in China. *Transactions of the Royal Society of Tropical Medicine and Hygiene* 92: 135–136 (1998)

Bradley DJ. Malaria—whence and whither? *In*: Malaria: waiting for the vaccine (Ed G.A.T. Targett). Wiley. Chichester. ISBN 0471 93100 4 (1991)

Bradley D, Coluzzi M. The Malaria Challenge After 100 Years of Malariology. *Parassitologia* 41: 1 – 3 (1999)

Breman JG, Mills A, Snow RW, Mulligan JA, Lengeler C, Mendis K, Sharp B, Morel C, Marchesini P, White N, Steketee R, Doumbo O Conquering Malaria (413–32). In Jamison DT, Breman JG, Measham AR, Alleyne G, Claeson M, Evans DB, Jha P, Mills A, Musgrove P (eds) Disease Control Priorities in developing Countries. *Oxford University Press and The Worldbank* (2006)

Brewster DR, Greenwood BM. Seasonal variation of paediatric diseases in The Gambia. *Annals of Tropical Paediatrics* 13: 133–46 (1993)

Brinkmann U, Brinkmann A. Malaria and health in Africa: the present situation and epidemiological trends. *Tropical Medicine and Parasitology* 42: 204–213 (1991)

Bruce-Chwatt LJ. History of malaria from prehistory to eradication. In: Wernsdorfer & McGregor (Eds.), Malaria – Principles and Practice of Malariology (pp. 1–60). *Churchill Livingstone*, London (1988)

Bruce-Chwatt L. Resurgence of malaria and its control. *Journal of Tropical Medicine Hygiene* 77 (supplement): 62–66 (1974)

Bruce-Chwatt L. Lessons learned from applied field research activities in Africa during the malaria eradication area. *Bulletin of the World Health Organization* 62 (supplement): 19–29 (1984)

Brun L, Sales S. Stage IV evaluation of four organophospho-rus insecticides applied at 0.2 gm/m to cotton mosquito nets. WHO mimeographed document, *WHO/VBC*, 76.630 (1976)

Brutus L, Watier L, Briand V, Hanitrasoamampionona V, Razanatsoarilala H, Cot M. Parasitic co-infections: does Ascaris lumbricoides protect against Plasmodium falciparum infection? *American Journal Tropical Medicine Hygiene* 75: 194–98 (2006)

Bugmann N. Le concept du paludisme, l'usage et l'efficacité in vivo de trois traitements traditionnels antipalustres dans la Région de Dori, Burkina Faso. *PhD thesis*, University of Basel (2000)

Buko Pharma-Kampagne. Malaria: Vom Oberrhein bis in die Tropen. ISSN 1618–4580. *Buko Pharma-Kampagne Bielefeld*, Deutschland (2010)

Burkot TR, Graves PM. Malaria, Babesiosis, Theileriosis and Related Diseases. In: Medical Entomology (Editors: Eldridge BF & Edman JD). *Kluwer Academic Publisher* (2000)

Calis JCJ, Phiri KS, Faragher EB, Brabin BJ, Bates I, Cuevas LE, de Haan RJ, Phiri AI, Malange P, Khoka M, Hulshof PJM, Lisette van Lieshout, Beld MG, Teo YY, Rockett KA, Richardson A, Kwiatkowski DP, Molyneux ME, Boele van Hensbroek M. Severe Malaria in Malawian children. *The New England Journal of Medicine* 358: 888–99 (2008)

Carme B. Low malaria mortality among children and high rates of *P. falciparum* inoculation: a Congolese reality in the 1980th. *Parasitology Today* 12: 206–8 (1996)

Carter R, Mendis KN. Evolutionary and historical aspects of the burden of malaria. *Clinical and Microbiological Reviews* 15:564–94 (2002)

CDI Study Group. Community-directed interventions for priority health problems in Africa: results of a multicountry study. *Bulletin of the World Health Organization* 88: 509–18 (2010)

Ceesay SJ, Casals-Pascual C, Erskine J, Anya SE, Duah NO, Fulford AJC, Sesay SSS, Abubakar I, Dunyo S, Sey O, Palmer A, Fofana M, Corrah T, Bojang KA, Whittle HC, Greenwood BM, Conway DJ. Changes in malaria indices between 1999 and 2007 in The Gambia: a retrospective analysis. *The Lancet* 372: 1545–54 (2008)

Chan M. Return to Alma-Ata. *The Lancet* 372: 865–66 (2008)

Chandramohan D, Owusu-Agyei S, Carneiro I, Awine T, Amponsa-Achiano K, Mensah N, Jaffar S, Baiden R, Hodgson A, Binka F, Greenwood B. Cluster randomised trial of intermittent preventive treatment for malaria in infants in area of high, seasonal transmission in Ghana. *BMJ* 331:727–733 (2005)

Chandre F, Darrier F, Manga L, Akogbeto M, Faye O, Mouchet J, Guillet P. Status of pyrethroid resistance in Anopheles gambiae sensu lato. *Bulletin of the World Health Organisation* 77:230–34 (1999)

Chareonviriyaphap T, Bangs MJ, Ratanatham S. Status of malaria in Thailand. *Southest Asian Journal of Tropical Medicine and Public Health* 31: 225–36 (2000)

Chen L, Evans T, Anand S, Boufford JI, Brown H, Chowdhury M, Cueto M, Dare L, Dussault G, Elzinga G, Fee E, Habte D, Hanvoravongchai P, Jacobs M, Kurowski C, Michael S, Pablos-Mendez A, Sewankambo N, Solimano G, Stilwell B, de Waal A, Wibulpolprasert S. Human resources for health: overcoming the crisis. *The Lancet* 364: 1984–90 (2004)

Chico RM, Chandramohan D. Quinine for the treatment of malaria in pregnancy. *The Lancet Infectious Diseases* 10: 140–41 (2010)

Chico RM, Pittrof R, Greenwood B, Chandramohan D. Azithromycin-chloroquine and the intermittent preventive treatment of malaria in pregnancy. *Malaria Journal* 7:255 (2008)

Chinkhumba J, Skarbinski J, Chilima B, Campbell C, Ewing V, Joaquin MS, Sande J, Ali D, Mathanga D. Comparative field performance and adherence to test results of four malaria rapid diagnostic tests among febrile patients more than five years of age in Blantyre, Malawi. *Malaria Journal* 9: 209 (2010)

Choi H, Breman J, Teutsch S, LiuS, Hightower A, Sexton J. The effectiveness of insecticide-impregnated bed nets in reducing cases of malaria infection: a meta-analysis of published results. *American Journal of Tropical Medicine and Hygiene* 52: 377–382 (1995)

Cissé B, Cheikh C, Boulanger D, Milet J, Bâ EH, Richardson K, Hallett R, Sutherland C, Simondon K, Simondon F, Alexander N, Gaye O, Targett G, Lines J, Greenwood B, Trape J. Seasonal intermittent preventive treatment with artesunate and sulfadoxine pyrimethamine prevents malaria in Senegalese children. *The Lancet* 367: 659–667 (2006)

Clarke SE, Jukes MCH, Njagi JK, Khasakhala L, Cundill B, Otido J, Crudder C, Estambale BBA, Brooker S. Effect of intermittent preventive treatment of malaria on health and education in schoolchildren: a cluster-randomised, double-blind, placebo-controlled trial. *The Lancet* 372: 127–38 (2008)

Clinton B. Keynote lecture. XVIII International AIDS Conference, Vienna, Austria, July 2010

Clyde D History of Medical Services of Tanganyika. Government Press, Dar es Salaam (1962)

Clyde D. Recent trends in the epidemiology and control of malaria. *Epidemiological Reviews* 9: 219–243 (1987)

Cockburn R, Newton PN, Agyarko KE, Akunyili D, Withe NJ. The Global Threat of Counterfeit Drugs: Why Industry and Government Must Communicate the Danger. *PLoS Medicine* 2:e100, 2005

Coleman M, Coleman M, Mabaso MLH, Mabuza AM, Kok G, Coetzee M, Durrheim DN. Household and microeconomoc factors associated with malaria in Mpumalanga, South Africa. *Transactions of the Royal Society of Tropical Medicine and Hygiene* 104: 143–47 (2010)

Collins WE, Barnwell JW. A hopeful beginning for malaria vaccines. *The New England Journal of Medicine* 359: 2599–2601 (2008)

Coll-Seck AM. A golden age for malaria research and innovation. *Malaria Journal* 7: S2 (2008)

Comoro C, Nsimba SED, Warsame M, Tomson G. Local understanding, perceptions and reported practices of mothers/guardians and health workers on childhood malaria in a Tanzanian district – implications for malaria control. *Acta Tropica* 87: 305–313 (2003)

Condraun JM, Ford N, Henkens M, Macé C, Kiddle-Monroe R, Pinel J. Substandard medicines in resource-poor settings: a problem that can no longer be ignored. *Tropical Medicine & International Health* 13: 1062–72 (2008)

Cornetto G, Ooms G, Starrs A, Zeitz P. A global fund for the health MDGs? *The Lancet* 373: 1500–02 (2009)

Coulibaly B, Zoungrana A, Mockenhaupt F, Schirmer H, Klose C, Mansmann U, Meissner P, Müller O. Strong gametocytocidal effect of methylene blue-based combination therapy against falciparum malaria: a randomised controlled trial. *PLoS One* 4 (5): e5318 (2009)

Crawley J, Chu C, Mtove G, Nosten F. Malaria in children. *The Lancet* 375: 1468–81 (2010)

Curtis CF, Mnzava AEP. Comparison of house spraying and insecticide-treated nets for malaria control. *Bulletin of the World Health Organisation* 78:1389–1401 (2000)

Curtis C, Maxwell C, Lemnge M, Kilama WL, Steketee RW, Hawley WA, Bergevin Y, Campbell CC, Sachs J, Teklehaimanot A, Ochola S, Guyatt H, Snow RW. Scaling-up coverage with insecticide-treated nets against malaria in Africa: who should pay? *The Lancet Infectious Diseases* 3: 304–7 (2003)

Dabiré RK, Diabaté A, Baldet T, Paré-Toé L, Guigemdé RT, Ouédraogo JB, Skovmand O. Personal protection of long-lasting ITNs in areas of Anopheles gambiae s.s. resistance to pyrethroids. *Malaria Journal* 5: 12 (2006)

Dabis F, Breman JG, Roisin AJ, Haba F, The ACSI CCCD Team Monitoring selective components of primary health care: methodology and community assessment of vaccination, diarrhoea and malaria practices in Conakry, Guinea. *Bulletin of the World Health Organization* 67, 675–684 (1989)

D'Alessandro U, Olaleye B, McGuire W, Langerock P, Bennett S, Aikins M, Thomson M, Cham K, CHAM B, Greenwood B. Mortality and morbidity from malaria in Gambian children after introduction of an impregnated bednet programme. *The Lancet* 345: 479–483 (1995)

D'Alessandro U, Langerock P, Bennett S, Francis N, Cham K, Greenwood B. The impact of a national impregnated bed net programme on the outcome of pregnancy in primigravidae in The Gambia. *Transactions of the Royal Society of Tropical Medicine and Hygiene* 90: 487–492 (1996)

D'Alessandro U. Existing antimalarial agents and malaria treatment strategies. Expert opinion in Pharmacotherapy 10: 1291–1306 (2009)

Danquah I, Coulibaly B, Meissner P, Petruschke I, Müller O, Mockenhaupt FP. Selection of pfmdr1 and pfcrt alleles in amodiaquine treatment failure in north-western Burkina Faso. *Acta Tropica* 114:123–27 (2010)

Das P, Horton R. Malaria elimination: worthy, challenging, and just possible. *The Lancet* 376: 1515–17 (2010)

De Alencar F, Cerutti C, Durlacher R, Boulos M, Alves F, Milhous W, Pang L. Atovaquone and proguanil for the treatment of malaria in Brazil. *Journal of Infectious Diseases* 175: 1544–1547 (1997)

Delacollette C, Van Der Stuyft P, Molima K. Using community health workers for malaria control: experience in Zaire. *Bulletin of the World Health Organization* 74: 423–430 (1996)

Deming M, Gayibor A, Murphy K, Jones T, Karsa T. Home treatment of febrile children with antimalarial drugs in Togo. *Bulletin of the World Health Organization* 67: 695–700 (1989)

Deressa W, Ali A, Enqusellassie F. Self-treatment of malaria in rural communities, Butajira, southern Ethiopia. *Bulletin of the World Health Organization* 81: 261–268 (2003)

De Sousa A, Salama P, Chopra M. Implementing intermittent preventive treatment in infants. *The Lancet* 375:121 (2010)

De Vries P, Dien T. Clinical pharmacology and therapeutic potential of artemisinin ande its derivates in the treatment of malaria. *Drugs* 52: 818–836 (1996)

Dhingra N, Jha P, Sharma VP, Cohen AA, Jotkar RM, Rodriguez PS, Bassani DG, Surrawera W, Laxminarayan R, Peto R, for the Million Deaths Study Collaborators. *The Lancet* 376: 1768–74 (2010)

Diallo DA, Cousens SN, Cuzin-Quattara N, Nebie I, Ilboudo-Sanogo E, Esposito F. Child mortality in a West African population protected with insecticide-treated curtains for a period of up to 6 years. *Bulletin of the World Health Organisation* 82: 85–91(2004)

Dicko A, Sagara I, Sissoko MS, Guindo O, Diallo AI, Kone M, Toure OB, Sacko M, Doumbo OK. Impact of intermittent preventive treatment with sulfadoxine-pyrimethamine targeting the transmission season on the incidence of clinical malaria inchildren aged 6 months to 10 years in Kambila, Mali. *American Journal of Tropical Medicine and Hygiene* 71 (Suppl. S4): 6 (2004)

Diesfeld HJ. Von Rudolf Virchow zu den Milleniums-Entwicklungszielen 2000. In: Razum, Zeeb & Laser (Eds.), Globalisierung – Gerechtigkeit – Gesundheit, Einführung in International Public Health (pp. 19–26). *Verlag Hans Huber* (2006)

Dondorp A, Nosten F, Stepniewska K, Day N, White N, South East Asian Ouinine Artesunate Malaria Trial (SEAQUAMAT) group. Artesunate versus quinine for treatment of severe falciparum malaria: a randomised trial. *The Lancet* 366: 717–25 (2005)

Dondorp AM, Nosten F, Yi P, Das D, Phyo AP, Tarning J, Lwin KM, Ariey F, Hanpithakpong W, Lee SJ, Ringwald P, Silamut K, Imwong M, Chotivanich K, Lim P, Herdman T, An SS, Yeung S, Singhasivanon P, Day NPJ, Lindegardh N, Socheat D, Nicholas J. White NJ. Artemisinin resistance in *Plasmodium falciparum* malaria. *The New England Journal of Medicine* 361: 455–467 (2009)

Dondorp AM, Fanello CI, Hendriksen ICE, Gomes E, Seni A, Chhaganlal KD, Bojang K, Olaosebikan R, Anunobi N, Maitland K, Kivaya E, Agbenyega T, Nguah SB, Evans J, Gesase S, Kahabuka C, Mtove G, Nadjm B, Deen J, Mwanga-Amumpaire J, Nansumba M, Karema C, Umulisa N, Uwimana A, Mokuolu OA, Adedoyin OT, Johnson WBR, Tshefu AK, Onyamboko MA, Sakulthaew T, Ngum WP, Silamut K, Stepniewska K, Woodrow CJ, Bethell D, Wills B, Oneko M, Peto TE, von Seidlein L, Da NPJ, White NJ, for the AQUAMAT group. Artesunate versus quinine in the treatment of severe falciparum malaria in African children (AQUAMAT): an open-label, randomised trial. *The Lancet* 376: 1647–57 (2010)

Donnelly MJ, Corbel V, Weetman D, Wilding CS, Williamson MS, Black WC. Does kdr genotype predict insecticide resistance phenotype in mosquitoes? *Trends in Parasitology* 25: 213–19 (2009)

Dopson MJ. The malarology centenary. *Parassitologia* 41: 21–32 (1999)

Druilhe P, Tall A, Sokhna C. Worms can worsen malaria: towards a new means to roll back malaria? *Trends in Parasitology* 21: 359–62 (2005)

Duffy & Mutabingwa. Rolling back a malaria epidemic in South Africa. *PLoS Medicine* 2: e368 (2005)

Elzinga G. Vertical-horizontal synergy of the health workforce. *Bulletin of the World Health Organization* 83: 4 (2005)

English M, Punt J, Mwangh I, McHugh K, Marsh K. Clinical overlap between malaria and severe pneumonia in African children in hospital. *Transactions of the Royal Society of Tropical Medicine and Hygiene* 90: 658–62 (1996)

Enserink M Global Health: Malaria Drugs, the Coca Cola Way. *Science* 322: 1174–76 (2008)

Etang J, Fondjo E, Chandre F, Morlais I, Brengues C, Nwane P, Chouaibou M, Ndjemai H, Simard F. First report of knockdown mutations in the malaria vector *Anopheles gambiae* from Cameroon. *American Journal of Tropical Medicine and Hygiene* 74: 795–97 (2006)

Evans DB, Adam T, Edejer TT, Lim SS, Cassels A, Evans TG. Achieving the millennium development goals for health: Time to reassess strategies for improving health in developing countries. *BMJ* 331: 1133–36 (2005)

Evans DB, Etienne C. Health systems financing and the path to universal coverage. *Bulletin of the World Health Organisation* 88: 402–3 (2010)

Farenhorst M, Knols BGJ, Thomas MB, Howard AFV, Takken W, Rowland M, N'Guessan R. Synergy in Efficacy of Fungal Entomopathogens and Permethrin against West African Insecticide-Resistant *Anopheles gambiae* Mosquitoes. *PloS One* 5 (8): e12081 (2010)

Feachem RGA, Sabot OJ. Global malaria control in the 21st century. *JAMA* 297: 2281–2284 (2007)

Feachem R, Sabot O. A new malaria eradication strategy. *The Lancet* 371: 1633–35 (2008)

Feachem RGA, Phillips AA. Malaria: 2 years in the fast lane. *The Lancet* 373: 1409–10 (2009)

Feachem RGA, Phillips AA, Hwang J, Cotter C, Wielgosz B, Greenwood BM, Sabot O, Rodriguez MH, Abeyasinghe RR, Ghebreyesus TA, Snow RW. Malaria Elimination Series I: Shrinking the malaria map – progress and prospects. *The Lancet* 376: 1566–78 (2010a)

Feachem RGA, Phillips AA, Targett GA, Snow RW. Call to action: priorities for malaria elimination. *The Lancet* 376: 1517–20 (2010b)

Fegan GW, Noor AM, Akhwale WS, Cousens S, Snow RW. Effect of expanded insecticide-treated bednet coverage on child survival in rural Kenya: a longitudinal study. *The Lancet* 370: 1035–1039 (2007)

Ferguson HM, Dornhaus A, Beeche A, Borgemeister C, Gottlieb M, Mulla MS, Gimnig JE, Fish D, Killeen GF. Ecology: A Prerequisite for Malaria Elimination and Eradication. *PLoS Medicine* 7:e1000303 (2010)

Field MG. The health crisis in the former Soviet Union: A report from the 'postwar' zone. *Social Science & Medicine* 41: 1469–78 (1995)

Fillinger U, Knols BG, Becker N (2003) Efficacy and efficiency of new *Bacillus thuringiensis* var. *israelensis* and *Bacillus sphaericus* formulations against afrotropical anophelines in western Kenya. *Tropical Medicine and International Health* 8(1): 37–47

Fillinger U, Sombroek H, Majambere S, van Loon E, Takken W, Lindsay SW Identifying the most productive breeding sites for malaria mosquitoes in The Gambia. *Malaria Journal* 8: 62 (2009a)

Fillinger U, Ndenga B, Githeko A, Lindsay SW. Integrated vector control with microbial larvicides and ITNs in western Kenya: a controlled trial. *Bulletin of the World Health Organization* 87: 655–65 (2009b)

Fontane RE, Pull JH, Payne D, Pradhan GD, Joshi GP, Pearson JA, Thymakis MK, Camacho MER Evaluation of fenitrothion for the control of malaria. *Bulletin of the World Health Organization* 56: 445–52 (1978)

French N, Nakiyingi J, Lugada E, Watera C, Whitworth JA, Gilks CF. Increasing rates of malarial fever with deteriorating immune status in HIV-1-infected Ugandan adults. *AIDS* 15(7):899–906 (2001)

Frey C, Traoré C, De Allegri M, Kouyaté B, Müller O. Compliance of young children with ITN protection in rural Burkina Faso. *Malaria Journal* 5: 69 (2006)

Fryatt R, Mills A, Nordstrom A. Financing of health systems to achieve the health MDGs in low-income countries. *The Lancet* 375: 419–26 (2010)

Gakidou E, Cowling K, Lozano R, Murray CJL. Increased educational attainment and its effect on child mortality in 175 countries between 1970 and 2009: a systematic analysis. *The Lancet* 376: 959–74 (2010)

Galinski MR, Barnwell JE. Monkey malaria kills four humans. *Trends in Parasitolgy* 25: 200–204 (2009)

Gallup JL, Sachs JD. The economic burden of malaria. *American Journal of Tropical Medicine and Hygiene* 64 (supplement): 85–96 (2001)

Garner P, Brabin B.: A review of randomized controlled trials of routine antimalarial drug prophylaxis during pregnancy in endemic malarious areas. *Bulletin of the World Health Organization* 72: 89–99 (1994)

Garner P, Gülmezoglu A: Prevention versus treatment for malaria in pregnant women Cochrane Review. In: *The Cochrane Library* Issue 3 Oxford: Update Software; (2001)

Garrett L, Chowdhury AMR, Pablos-Méndez A. All for universal health coverage. *The Lancet* 374: 1294–99 (2009)

Gerstl S, Dunkley S, Mukhtar A, Maes P, De Smet M, Baker S, Maikere J. Long-lasting ITN usage in eastern Sierra Leone – the success of free distribution. *Tropical Medicine & International Health* 15: 480–88 (2010)

Ghebreyesus TA, Haile M, Witten KH, Getachew A, Yohannes AM, Yohannes M, Teklehaimanot HD, Lindsay SW, Byass P. Incidence of malaria among children living near dams in northern Ethiopia: community based incidence survey. *BMJ* 319: 663–6 (1999)

Ghebreyesus TA. The Global Fund: replenishment and redefinition. *The Lancet* 376: 416–17 (2010a)

Ghebreyesus TA. Achieving the health MDGs: country ownership in four steps. *The Lancet* 376: 1127–28 (2010b)

Gies S. Preventing malaria in pregnancy by health promotion and intermittent preventive treatment: a community-based intervention in rural Burkina Faso. PhD Thesis, Institute of Tropical Medicine, *Antwerp University* (2009)

Gilks CF, Crowley S, Ekpin R, Gove S, Perriens J, Souteyrand Y, Sutherland D, Vitoria M, Guerma T, De Cock K. The WHO public-health approach to antiretroviral treatment against HIV in resource-limited settings. *The Lancet* 368: 505–10 (2006)

Gilles H, Warrell D. Bruce-Chwatt's Essential Malariology. Boston: *Little, Brown and Company* (1993)

Gilles H.: Historical outline. In: Bruce-Chwatt's Essential Malariology. Edited by Gilles and Warrell. Boston: *Little, Brown and Company* (1993)

Gimnig JE, Slutsker L. House screening for malaria control. *The Lancet* 374: 954–55 (2009)

Global Fund. www.theglobalfund.org, *accessed 15.10.2010* (2010)

Gomes M, Salazar N. Chemotherapy: principles in practice – a case study of The Philippines. *Social Science & Medicine* 30, 789–796 (1990)

Gomes MF, Faiz MA, Gyapong JO, Warsame M, Agbenyega T, Babiker A, Baiden F, Yunus EB, Binka F, Clerk C, Folb P, Hassan R, Hossain MA, Kimbute O, Kitua A, Krishna S, Makasi C, Mensah N, Mrango Z, Olliaro P, Peto R, Peto TJ, Rahman MR, Ribeiro I, Samad R, White NJ. Pre-referral rectal artesunate to prevent death and disability in severe malaria: a placebo-controlled trial. *The Lancet* 373: 557–66 (2009)

Gonzales JO, Kroeger A, Avina AI, Pabon E. Wash resistance of insecticide-treated materials. *Transactions of the Royal Society of Tropical Medicine and Hygiene* 96:370–75 (2002)

Goodman CA, Coleman PG, Mills AJ. Cost-effectiveness of malaria control in sub-Saharan Africa. *The Lancet* 354: 378–85 (1999)

Gosling RD, Gesase S, Mosha JF, Carneiro I, Hashim R, Lemnge M, Mosha FW, Greenwood B, Chandramohan D. Protective efficacy and safety of three antimalarial regimens for intermittant preventive treatment for malaria in infants: a randomised, double-blind, placebo-controlled trial. *The Lancet* 374: 1521–32 (2009)

Gostin L. The unconscionable health gap: a global plan for justice. *The Lancet* 375: 1504–5 (2010)

Gramiccia G, Beales PF. The recent history of malaria control and eradication. In: Wernsdorfer & McGregor (Eds.), Malaria – Principles and Practice of Malariology (pp. 1335–1378). *Churchill Livingstone, London* (1988)

Graves PM, Richards FO, Ngondi J, Emerson PM, Shargie EB, Endeshaw T, Ceccato P, Ejigsemahu Y, Mosher AW, Hailemariam A, Zerihun M, Teferi T, Ayele

B, Mesele A, Yohannes G, Tilahun A, Gebre T. Individual, household and environmental risk factors for malaria infection in Amhara, Oromia and SNNP regions of Ethiopia. *Transactions of the Royal Society of Tropical Medicine and Hygiene* 103: 1211–20 (2009)

Greenwood B, Bradley A, Greenwood A, Byass P, Jammeh K, Marsh S, Tulloch F, Oldfield F, Hayes R. Mortality and morbidity from malaria among children in a rural area of The Gambia. *Transactions of the Royal Society of Tropical Medicine and Hygiene* 81: 478–486 (1987)

Greenwood B, Greenwood A, Bradley A, Snow R, Byass P, Hayes R, N'Jie A. Comparison of two strategies for control of malaria within a primary health care programme in The Gambia. *The Lancet* I: 1121–1127 (1988)

Greenwood B, Greenwood A, Snow R, Byass P, Bennett S, Hatib-N'Jie A. The effects of malaria chemoprophylaxis given by traditional birth attendants on the course and outcome of pregnancy. *Transactions of the Royal Society of Tropical Medicine and Hygiene* 83: 589–594 (1989)

Greenwood B. Impact of culture and environmental changes on epidemiology and control of malaria and babesiosis: The microepidemiology of malaria and its importance to malaria control. *Transactions of the Royal Society of Tropical Medicine and Hygiene* 83 (supplement): 25–29 (1989)

Greenwood A, Bradley A, Byass P, Greenwood B, Snow R, Bennett S, Hatib-N'JIE, A. Evaluation of a PHC programme in The Gambia. I The impact of trained traditional birth attendants on the outcome of pregnancy. *Journal of Tropical Medicine and Hygiene* 93: 58–66 (1990)

Greenwood B. Malaria transmission and vector control. *Parasitology Today* 13: 90–92 (1997)

Greenwood B. Malaria mortality and morbidity in Africa. *Bulletin of the World Health Organization* 77: 617–8 (1999)

Greenwood B. What can the residents of malaria endemic countries do to protect themselves against malaria? Parassitologia 41: 295–9 (1999)

Greenwood BM, Bojang K, Whitty CJM, Targett GAT. Seminar Series: Malaria. *The Lancet* 365: 1487–98 (2005)

Greenwood BM. Review: Intermittent preventive treatment – a new approach to the prevention of malaria in children in areas with seasonal malaria transmission. *Tropical Medicine & International Health* 11: 983–91 (2006)

Greenwood B. Intermittent preventive antimalarial treatment in infants. *Clinical Infectious Diseases* 45: 6–28 (2007)

Greenwood BM, Fidock DA, Kyle DE, Kappe SHI, Alonso PL, Collins FH, Duffy PE Malaria: progress, perils, and prospects for eradication. *The Journal of Clinical Investigation* 118: 1266–76 (2008)

Griffin JT, Hollingsworth TD, Okell LC, Churcher TS, White M, Hinsley W, Bousema T, Drakeley CJ, Ferguson NM, Basa'n~ ez1 MG, Ghani1 AC. Reducing Plasmodium falciparum Malaria Transmission in Africa: A Model-Based Evaluation of Intervention Strategies. *PLoS Medicine* 7: e1000324 (2010)

Grimwade K, French N, Mbatha DD, Zungu DD, Dedicoat M, Gilks CF. Childhood malaria in a region of unstable transmission and high human immunodeficiency virus prevalence. *Pediatric Infecious Diseases J* 22(12):1057–63 (2003)

Guerra CA, Gikandi PW, Tatem AJ, Noor AM, Smith DL, Hay SI, Snow RW. The Limits and Intensity of *Plasmodium falciparum* Transmission: Implications for Malaria Control and Elimination Worldwide. *PloS Medicine* 5: 2, e38 (2008)

Guerra CA, Howes RE, Patil AP, Gething PW, Boeckel TPV, Temperley WH, Kabaria CW, Tatem AJ, Manh BH, Elyazar IRF, Baird JK, Snow RW, Hay SI. The International Limits and Population at Risk of *Plasmodium vivax* Transmission in 2009. *PloS Neglected Tropical Diseases* 4: 8, e774 (2010)

Gusmao R. Overview of malaria control in the Americas. *Parassitologia* 41: 355–60 (1999)

Guttmann P, Ehrlich P. Über die Wirkung des Methylenblau bei Malaria. *Berliner Klinische Wochenschrift* 39: 953–956 (1891)

Gyapong JO, Gyapong M, Yellu N, Anakwah K, Amofah G, Bockarie M, Adjei S. Integration of control of neglected tropical diseases into health-care systems: challeneges and opportunities. The Lancet 375: 160–65 (2010)

Haines A, Sanders D, Lehmann U, Rowe AK, Lawn JE, Jan S, Walker DG, Bhutta Z. Achieving child survival goals: potential contribution of community health workers. *The Lancet* 369: 2121–31 (2007)

Hall KA, Newton PN, Green MD, de Veij M, Vandenabeele P, Pizzanelli D, Mayxay M, Dondorp A, Fernandez F. Characterization of counterfeit artesunate antimalarial tablets from southeast Asia. *American Journal of Tropical Medicine and Hygiene* 75:804–811 (2006)

Hamer DH, Ndhlovu M, Zurovac D, Fox M, Yeboah-Antwi K, Chanda P, Sipilinyambe N, Simon JL, Snow RW. Improved Diagnostic Testing and Malaria Treatment Practices in Zambia. *JAMA* 297: 2227–31 (2007)

Hammer GP, Somé F, Müller O, Kynast-Wolf G, Kouyaté B, Becher H. Pattern of cause-specific childhood mortality in a malaria endemic area of Burkina Faso. *Malaria Journal* 5: 47 (2006)

Hansen K, Kikumbih N, Armstrong-Schellenberg J. Cost-effectiveness of social marketing of insecticide-treated mosquito nets for malaria control in the United Republic of Tanzania. *Bulletin of the World Health Organisation* 81: 269–76 (2003)

Hanson S, Schwartlander B, Walker N. HIV/AIDS control in sub-Saharan Africa. *Science* 294(5542): 521–3 (2001)

Harries AD, Schouten EJ, Libamba E. Scaling up antiretroviral treatment in resource-poor settings. *The Lancet* 367: 1870–72 (2006)

Harris I, Sharrock WW, Bain LM, Gray KA, Bobogare A, Boaz L, Lilley K, Krause D, Vallely A, Johnson ML, Gatton ML, Shanks GD, Cheng Q. A large proportion of asymptomatic *Plasmodium* infections with low and sub-microscopic parasite densities in the low transmission setting of Temotu Province, Solomon Islands: challenges for malaria diagnostics in an elimination setting. *Malaria Journal* 9:254 (2010)

Harrison G. Mosquitoes, malaria and man: a history of the hostilities since 1880. *Dutton EP, New York, USA* (1978)

Hartgers FC, Yazdanbakhsh M. Co-infection of helminths and malaria: modulation of the immune responses to malaria. *Parasite Immunology* 28: 497–506 (2006)

Hastings IM, Bray PG, Ward SA. A requiem for chloroquine. *Science* 298: 74–75 (2002)

Hastings IM, Korenromp EL, Bloland PB. The anatomy of a malaria disaster: drug policy choice and mortality in African children. *The Lancet Infectious Diseases* 7: 739–48 (2007)

Hawass Z, Gad YZ, Ismail S. Ancestry and pathology in King Tutankhamun's family. *JAMA* 303: 638–47 (2010)

Hawley WA, Ter Kuile FO, Steketeee RS. Implications of the western Kenya permethrin-treated bed net study for policy, program implementation, and future research. *American Journal of Tropical Medicine and Hygiene* 68 (supplement): 168–73 (2003)

Hay SI, Omumbo JA, Craig MH, Snow RW. Earth observation, geographic information systems and Plasmodium falciparum malaria in sub-Saharan Africa. Advances in Parasitology 47:173–215 (2000)

Hay SI, Rogers DJ, Toomer JF, Snow RW. Annual Plasmodium falciparum entomological inoculation rates (EIR) across Africa: literature survey, Internet access and review. *Transactions of the Royal Society of Tropical Medicine and Hygiene* 94: 113–27 (2000)

Hay IH, Gething PW, Snow RW. India's invisible malaria burden. *The Lancet* 376: 1716–17 (2010)_

Hay SI, Guerra CA, Tatem AJ, Noor AM, Snow RW. The global distribution and population at risk of malaria: past, present, and future. *The Lancet Infectious Diseases* 4: 327–36 (2004)

Hay SI, Smith DL, Snow RW. Measuring malaria endemicity from intense to interrupted transmission. *The Lancet Infectious Diseases* 8: 369–78 (2008)

Helitzer-Allen DL, McFarland DA, Wirima JJ, Macheso AP. Malaria chemoprophylaxis compliance in pregnant women: a cost effectiveness analysis of alternative interventions. *Social Science and Medicine* 36:403–407 (1993)

Hewitt K, Steketee R, Mwapasa V, Whitworth J, French N. Interactions between HIV and malaria in non-pregnant adults: evidence and implications. *AIDS* 20: 1993–2004 *(2006)*

Hien T, White N. Qinghaosu. *The Lancet* 603–608 (1993)

Hien T, Day N, Phu N, Mai N, Chau T, Loc P, Sinh D, Chuong L, Vinh H, Waller D, Chir B, Peto T, White N. A controlled trial of artemether or quinine in Vietnamese adults with severe falciparum malaria. *The New England Journal of Medicine* 335: 76–83 (1996)

Hill AVS. Malaria resistance genes: a natural selection. *Transactions of the Royal Society of Tropical Medicine and Hygiene* 86: 225–26 (1992)

Hoffman S. Save the children. *Nature* 430: 940–41 (2004)

Holtz TH, Kachur SP, Marum LH, Mkandala C, Chizani N, Roberts JM, Macheso A, Parise ME. Care seeking behaviour and treatment of febrile illness in children aged less than five years: a household survey in Blantyre District, Malawi. *Transactions of the Royal Society of Tropical Medicine and Hygiene* 97: 491–7 (2003)

Hongoro C, McPake B: How to bridge the gap in human resources for health. *The Lancet* 364: 1451–6 (2004)

Huailu C, Wen Y, Wuanmin K, Chongyl L. Large-scale spraying of bed nets to control mosquito vectors and malaria in Sichuan, China. *Bulletin of the World Health Organization* 73: 321–328 (1995)

Hudson A. Atovaquone – a novel broad-spectrum anti-infective drug. *Parasitology Today* 9: 66–68 (1993)

Hutton G. Is the jury still out on the impact of user fees in Africa? A review of the evidence from selected countries on user fees and determinants of health service utilisation. *East African Medical Journal* 81: 45–60 (2004)

Ijumba JN, Lindsay SW. Impact of irrigation on malaria in Africa: paddies paradox. *Medical and Veterinary Entomology* 15(1):1–11 (2001)

Ilboudo-Sanogo E, Cuzin-Ouattara N, Diallo DA, Cousens SN, Esposito F, Habluetzel A, Sanon S, Ouédraogo AP. Insecticide-treated materials, mosquito adaptation and mass effect: entomological observations after five years of vector control in Burkina Faso. *Transactions of the Royal Society of Tropical Medicine and Hygiene* 95: 353–60 (2001)

INDEPTH-Network. Population and health in developing countries – Population, Health, and Survival at INDEPTH sites. Ottawa: International Development Research Centre (2002)

INDEPTH. Research proposal for a phase IV safety and effectiveness platform. Accra, Ghana (2010)

International Artemisinin Study Group Artesunate combinations for treating uncomplicated malaria: a prospective individual patient data meta-analysis. *The Cochrane Library* Issue 2 Oxford (2009)

Jaffar S, Leach A, Greenwood A, Jepson A, Müller O, Ota M, Bojang K, Obaro S, Greenwood B. Changes in the pattern of infant and childhood mortality in Upper River Division, The Gambia, from 1989 to 1993. *Tropical Medicine and International Health* 2: 28–37 (1997)

Källander K, Nsungwa-Sabiiti J. Home-based management of malaria in the era of urbanisation. *The Lancet* 373: 1582–1584 (2009)

Kalk A, Paul FA, Grabosch E. Paying for performance in Rwanda: does it pay off? *Tropical Medicine & International Health 15*: 182–90 (2010)

Kamal-Yanni M. Affordable medicines facility for malaria: reasonable or rash? *The Lancet* 375: 121 (2010)

Kaseje D, Sempebwa E, Spencer H. Malaria chemoprophylaxis to pregnant women provided by community health workers in Saradidi, Kenya. I. Reasons for non-acceptance. *Annals of Tropical Medicine and Parasitology* 81: 77–82 (1987)

Kazatchkine MD. Increased resources for the Global Fund, but pledges fall short of expected demand. *The Lancet* 376: 1439–40 (2010)

Kean B. Chloroquine-resistant falciparum malaria from Africa. *JAMA* 241: 395 (1979)

Kelly-Hope LA, McKenzie FE. The multiplicity of malaria transmission: a review of entomological inoculation rate measurements and methods across sub-Saharan Africa. *Malaria Journal* 8: 19 (2008)

Kelly-Hope LA, Ranson H, Hemingway J. Lessons from the past: managing insecticide resistance in malaria control and eradication programmes. *The Lancet Infectious Diseases* 8: 387–89 (2008)

Kerber J, de Graft-Johnson JE, Bhutta ZA, Okong P, Starrs A, Lawn JE. Continuum of care for maternal, newborn, and child health: from slogan to service delivery. *The Lancet* 317: 1358–69 (2007)

Keusch GT, Kilama WL, Moon S, Szlezak NA, Michaud CM. The Global Health System: Linking Knowledge with Action – Learning from Malaria. *PLoS Medicine* 7: e1000179 (2010)

Kidane G, Morrow RH: Teaching mothers to provide home treatment of malaria in Tigray, Ethiopia: a randomised trial. *The Lancet* 356:550–55 (2000)

Kirby MJ, Ameh D, Bottomley C, Green C, Jawara M, Milligan PJ, Snell PC, Conway DJ, Lindsay SW. Effect of two different house screening interventions on exposure to malaria vectors and on anaemia in children in The Gambia: a randomised controlled trial. *The Lancet* 374: 998–1009 (2009)

Kitua AY, Smith T, Alonso PL, Masanja H, Menendez C, Urassa, H, Kimario J, Tanner M. *Plasmodium falciparum* malaria in the first year of life in an area of intense and perennial transmission. *Tropical Medicine and International Health* 1: 475–484 (1996)

Kleinschmidt I, Sharp B, Benavente LE, Schwabe C, Torrez M, Kuklinski J, Morris N, Raman J, Carter J. Reduction in infection with Plasmodium falciparum one year after the introduction of malaria control interventions on Bioko Island, Equatorial Guinea. *American Journal of Tropical Medicine and Hygiene* 74: 972–78 (2006)

Kleinschmidt I, Torrez M, Schwabe C, Benavente L, Seocharan I, Jituboh D, Nseng G, Brian Sharp. Factors influencing the effectiveness of malaria control in Bioko Island, Equatorial Guinea. *Malaria Journal* 76: 1027–32 (2007)

Kleinschmidt I, Schwabe C, Benavente L, Torrez M,. Ridl MC, Segura JL, Ehmer P, Nchama GN. Marked Increase in Child Survival after Four Years of Intensive Malaria Control. *American Journal of Tropical Medicine and Hygiene.* 80: 882–88 (2009)

Kober K, Van Damme W. Scaling up access to antiretroviral treatment in southern Africa: who will do the job? *The Lancet* 364: 103–7 (2004)

Korenromp EL, Williams BG, de Vlas SJ, Gouws E, Gilks CF, Ghys PD, Nahlen BL. Malaria attributable to the HIV-1 epidemic, sub-Saharan Africa. *Emerging Infectious Diseases Journal* 11: 1410–1419 (2005)

Korenromp EL, Williams BG, Gouws E, Dye C, Snow RW. Measurement of trends in childhood malaria mortality in Africa: an assessment of progress toward targets based on verbal autopsy. *The Lancet Infectious Diseases* 3: 349–358 (2003)

Kouyaté B, Sie A, Yé M, De Allegri M, Müller O. The great failure of malaria control in Africa: a district perspective from Burkina Faso. *PLoS Medicine* 4 (6): e127 (2007)

Kouyaté B, Somé F, Jahn A, Coulibaly B, Eriksen J, Sauerborn R, Gustafsson L, Tomson G, Becher H, Müller O. Process and effects of a community intervention on malaria in rural Burkina Faso: randomized controlled trial. *Malaria Journal* 7: 50 (2008)

Krause G, Sauerborn R. Community-effectiveness of care – the example of malaria treatment in rural Burkina Faso. *Annals of Tropical Paediatrics* 7: 99–106 (2000)

Kröger A, Skovmand O, Phan QC, Boewono DT. Combined field and laboratory evaluation of a long-term impregnated bednet, PermaNet. *Transactions of the Royal Society of Tropical Medicine and Hygiene* 98: 152–155 (2004)

Külker R, Prytherch H, Ruppel A, Müller O. Gesundheit für alle – aber ohne Personal? *Deutsches Ärzteblatt* 107:927–29 (2010)

Kynast-Wolf G, Hammer GP, Müller O, Kouyaté B, Becher H. Season of death, and of birth, predict patterns of mortality in Burkina Faso. *International Journal of Epidemiology* 34: 1–9 (2005)

Lagarde M, Palmer N. The impact of user fees on health service utilization in low- and middle-income countries: how strong is the evidence? *Bulletin of the World Health Organization* 86: 839–848 (2008).

Laufer MK, Thesing PC, Eddington ND, Masonga R, Dzinjalamala FK, Takala SL, Taylor TE, Plowe CV. Return of chloroquine antimalarial efficacy in Malawi. *The New England Journal of Medicine* 355: 1959–66 (2006)

Lawn JE, Rohde J, Rifkin S, Were M, Paul VK, Chopra M. Alma-Ata 30 years on: revolutionary, relevant, and time to revitalize. *The Lancet* 372: 917–27 (2008)

Lee K, Harmer A. Editorial: Ten years of the Global Alliance for Vaccines and Immunisation. *BMJ* 340: c2004 (2010)

Lee PW, Liu CT, do Rosario VE, de Sousa B, Rampao HS, Shaio MF. Potential threat of malaria epidemics in a low transmission area, as exemplified by Sao Tome and Principe *Malaria Journal* 9: 264 (2010)

Lell B, Luckner D, Ndjave M, Scott T, Kremsner P. Randomised placebo-controlled study of atovaquone plus proguanil for malaria prophylaxis in children. *The Lancet* 351: 709–713 (1998)

Lemma H, Byass P, Desta A, Bosman A, Costanzo G, Toma L, Fottrell E, Marrast A, Ambachew Y, Getachew A, Mulure N, Morrone A, Bianchi A, Barnabas GA. Deploying artemether-lumefantrine with rapid testing in Ethiopian communities: impact on malaria morbidity, mortality and healthcare resources. *Tropical Medicine and International Health.* 241–50 (2010)

Lengeler C, Snow R. From efficacy to effectiveness: Insecticide treated bed nets in Africa. *Bulletin of the World Health Organization* 74: 325–32 (1996)

Lengeler C. Insecticide treated bed nets and curtains for preventing malaria (Cochrane Review). In: *The Cochrane Library*. Oxford: Update Software (2004)

Leonard L. Where there is no state: household strategies for the management of illness in Chad. *Social Science and Medicine* 61:229–243 (2005)

Lepes T. Present status of the global malaria eradication programme and prospects for the future. *Journal of Tropical Medicine and Hygiene* 77 (supplement) 47–53 (1974)

Lindblade KA, Eisele TP, Gimnig JE, Alaii JA, Odhiambo F, ter Kuile FO, Hawley WA, Wannemuehler KA, Phillips-Howard PA, Rosen DH, Nahlen BL, Terlouw DJ, Adazu K, Vulule JM, Slutsker L. Sustainability of reductions in malaria transmission and infant mortality in western Kenya with use of insecticide-treated bednets 4 to 6 years of follow – up. *JAMA* 291: 2571–80 (2004)

Lindblade KA, Dotson E, Hawley WA. Evaluation of long-lasting insecticidal nets after 2 years of household use. *Tropical Medicine & International Health* 10: 1141–50 (2005)

Lindsay SW, Wilkins HA, Zidler HA, Daly RJ, Petrarca V, Byasi P. Ability of Anopheles gambiae to transmit malaria during the dry and wet seasons in an area of irrigated rice cultivation in The Gambia. *Journal of Tropical Medicine and Hygiene* 94: 313–14 (1991)

Lindsay SW, Alonso PL, Amstrong Shellenberg JRM, Hemingway J, Thomas PJ, Shenton FC, Greenwood BM. A malaria control trial using insecticide-treated bed nets and targeted chemoprophylaxis in a rural area of The Gambia, West Africa. 3. Entomological characteristics of the study area. *Transactions of the Royal Society of Tropical Medicine and Hygiene* 87 Supplement 2: 19–23 (1993)

Lines J, Lengeler C, Cham K. Scaling-up and sustaining ITN coverage in Africa. *The Lancet Infectious Diseases* 3: 466 (2003)

Lines J, Schapira A, Smith T. Tackling malaria today. *BMJ* 337: 435–37 (2008)

Liu W, Li Y, Learn GH, Rudicell RS, Robertson JD, Keele BF, Ndjango JBN, Sanz CM, Morgan DB, Locatelli S, Gonder MK, Kranzusch PJ, Walsh PD, Delaporte E, Mpoudi-Ngole E, Georgiev AV, Muller MN, Shaw GM, Peeters M, Sharp PM, Rayner JC, Hahn BH. Origin of the human malaria parasite *Plasmodium falciparum* in gorillas. *Nature* 467: 420–25 (2010)

Loewenberg S. The US President's malaria Initiative: 2 years on. *The Lancet* 370: 1893–94 (2007)

Looareesuwan S, Viravan C, Webster H, Kyle D, Hutchinson D, Canfield C. Clinical studies of atovaquone, alone or in combination with other antimalarial drugs, for treatment of acute uncomplicated malaria in Thailand. *American Journal of Tropical Medicine and Hygiene* 54: 62–66 (1996)

Lu C, Schneider MT, Gubbins P, Leach-Kemon K, Murray JCJL. Public financing of health in developing countries: a cross-national systematic analysis. *The Lancet* 375: 1375–87 (2010)

Lucas AO. Human resources for health in Africa. *BMJ* 331: 1037–40 (2005)

Mabaso MLH, Sharp B, Lengeler C. Historical review of malaria control in southern African with emphasis on the use of indoor residual house-spraying. *Tropical Medicine & International Health* 9: 846–56 (2004)

MacDonald G. The economic importance of malaria in Africa. WHO/MAL/60, Afr/Mal/Conf. 16. World Health Organisation, Geneva (1950)

Marmot M, Friel S, Bell R, Houweling TAJ, Taylor S. Closing the gap in a generation: health equity through action on the social determinants of health. *The Lancet* 372: 1661–69 (2008)

Marsh K, Forster D, Waruiru C, Mwangi, Winstanley M, Marsh V, Newton C, Winstanley P, Warn P, Peshu N, Pasvol G, Snow R. Indicators of Life-Threatening Malaria in African Children. *The New England Journal of Medicine* 332:1399–1404 (1995)

Marsh K. Malaria disaster in Africa. *The Lancet* 352: 924 (1998)

Marsh K. Research priorities for malaria elimination. *The Lancet* 376: 1626–27 (2010)

Matowe L, Adeyi O. The quest for universal access to effective malaria treatment: how can the AMFm contribute? *Malaria Journal* 9: 274 (2010)

Maxwell CA, Msuya E, Sudi M, Njunwa KJ, Carneiro IA, Curtis CF. Effect of community-wide use of insecticide-treated nets for 3–4 years on malaria morbidity in Tanzania. *Tropical Medicine & International Health* 7: 1003–8 (2002)

McCombie S. Treatment seeking for malaria: a review and suggestions for future research. Resource paper No. 2. TDR/SER/RP/94.1, UBDP/WORLD BANK/WHO – TDR (1994)

McCombie SC. Self-treatment for malaria: the evidence and methodological issues. *Health Policy and Planning* 17: 333–344 (2002)

McCoy D, Kembhavi G, Patel J, Luintel A. The Bill & Melinda Gates Foundation's grant-making programme for global health. *The Lancet* 373: 1645–53 (2009)

McDermott J, Slutsker L, Steketee W, Wirima J, Breman J, Heymann D. Prospective assessment of mortality among a cohort of pregnant women in rural Malawi. *American Journal of Tropical Medicine and Hygiene* 55 (supplement): 66–70 (1996)

McGregor IA. Epidemiology of malaria in pregnancy. *American Journal of Tropical Medicine and Hygiene* 33: 517–525 (1984)

MEG. The Malaria Elimination Group: Scope and Summary of First Meeting Santa Cruz, California, March 23 – 26. *Malaria Journal* (2008)

Meissner PE, Mandi G, Witte S, Coulibaly B, Mansmann U, Rengelshausen J, Schiek W, Jahn A, Sanon M, Tapsoba T, Walter-Sack I, Mikus G, Burhenne J, Riedel KD, Schirmer H, Kouyaté B, Müller O. Safety of the methylene blue plus chloroquine combination in the treatment of uncomplicated falciparum malaria in young children of Burkina Faso. *Malaria Journal* 4: 45 (2005)

Meissner PE, Mandi G, Coulibaly B, Witte S, Tapsoba T, Mansmann U, Rengelshausen J, Schiek W, Jahn A, Walter-Sack I, Mikus G, Burhenne J, Riedel KD, Schirmer RH, Kouyaté B, Müller O. Methylene blue for malaria in Africa: results from a dose-finding study in combination with chloroquine. *Malaria Journal* 5: 84 (2006)

Meissner P, Mandi G, Mockenhaupt F, Witte S, Coulibaly B, Mansmann U, Frey C, Schirmer RH, Müller O. Marked differences in the prevalence of chloroquine resistance between urban and rural communities in Burkina Faso. *Acta Tropica* 105: 81–86 (2008)

Mendis K, Sina BJ, Marchesini P, Carter R. The neglected burden of *Plasmodium vivax* malaria. *American Journal of Tropical Medicine and Hygiene* 64: 97–106 (2001)

Mendis K, Rietveld A, Warsame M, Bosman A, Greenwood B, Wernsdorfer WH. From malaria control to elimination: The WHO perspective. *Tropical Medicine & International Health* 14: 802–09 (2009)

Menendez C: Malaria during Pregnancy: a priority area of malaria research and control. *Parasitology Today* 11:178–183 (1995)

Menendez C, Kahigiwa E, Hirt R, Vounatsou P, Aponte J, Font F, Acosta C, Schellenberg D, Galindo C, Kimario J, Urassa H, Brabin B, Smith T, Kitua A, Tanner M, Alonso P. Randomized placebo-controlled trial of iron supplementation and malaria chemoprophylaxis for prevention of severe anaemia and malaria in Tansania. *The Lancet* 350: 844–850 (1997)

Menon A, Snow R, Byass P, Greenwood B, Hayes R, N'JIE A. Sustained protection against mortality and morbidity from malaria in rural Gambian children by chemoprophylaxis given by village health workers. *Transactions of the Royal Society of Tropical Medicine and Hygiene* 84: 768–772 (1990)

Meshnik SR, Taylor TE, Kamchonwongpaisan S. Artemisinin and the antimalarial endoperoxides: from herbal remedy to targeted chemotherapy. *Microbiological Reviews* 60: 301–15 (1996)

Meshnik SR Why does quinine still work after 350 years of use? *Parasitology Today* 13 (3): 89–90 (1997)

Mills A. Vertical vs horizontal health programmes in Africa: Idealism, pragmatism, resources and efficiency. *Social Science & Medicine* 17: 1971–81 (1983)

Mmbando BP, Vestergaard LS, Kitu AY, Lemnge MM, Theander TG, Lusingu JP. A progressive declining in the burden of malaria in north-eastern Tanzania. *Malaria Journal* 9: 216 (2010)

Modiano D. Petrarca V, Sirima B, Nebie I, Diallo D, Esposito F, Coluzzi M. Different response fo *Plasmodium falciparum* malaria in West African svmpatric ethnic groups. *Proceedings of the National Academy of Sciences of the United States of America* 93: 13206–2 11 (1996)

Modiano D, Sirima BS, Sawadogo A, Sanou I, Pare J, Konate A, Pagnoni F. Severe malaria in Burkina Faso: influence of age and transmission level on clinical presentation. *American Journal of Tropical Medicine and Hygiene* 59: 539–542 (1998)

Molineux L, Gramiccia G. The Garki Project. ISBN 92 4 156061 4. WHO/Geneva (1980)

Molyneux ME, Taylor TE, Wirima JJ & Harper G. Clinical features and prognostic indicators in paediatric cerebral malaria: a study of 131 comatose Malawian children. *Quarterly Journal of Medicine* 71: 441–459(1989)

Molyneux CS, Mung'ala-Odera V, Harpham T, Snow RW. Maternal responses to childhood fevers: a comparison of rural and urban residents in costal Kenya. *Tropical Medicine & International Health* 4, 836–845 (1999)

Molyneux DH. Patterns of change in vector-borne diseases. Annals of Tropical Medicine and Parasitology 91:827–39 (1997)

Molyneux DH, Hotez PJ, Fenwick A, Newman RD, Greenwood B, Sachs J. Neglected tropical diseases and the Global Fund. *The Lancet* 373: 296–97 (2009)

Moonen B, Cohen JM, Snow RW, Slutsker L, Drakeley C, Smith DL, Abeyasinghe RR, Rodriguez MH, Maharaj R, Tanner M, Targett G. Malaria Elimination Series III: Operational strategies to achieve and maintain malaria elimination. *The Lancet* 376: 1592–1603 (2010)

Morel CM, Lower JA, Evans DB. Cost-effectiveness analysis of strategies to combat malaria in developing countries. *BMJ* 331: 1299–1306 (2005)

Msellem MI, Mårtensson A, Rotllant G, Bhattarai A, Strömberg J, Kahigwa E, Garcia M, Max Petzold M, Peter Olumese P, Abdullah Ali A, Anders Björkman A. Influence of Rapid Malaria Diagnostic Tests on Treatment and Health Outcome in Fever Patients, Zanzibar—A Crossover Validation Study *PLOS Medicine* 6:e1000070 (2009)

Mugisha F, Kouyaté B, Gbangou A, Sauerborn R. Examining out of pocket expenditure on health care in Nouna, Burkina Faso: implications for health policy. Tropical *Medicine & International Health* 7:187–96 (2002)

Müller O, Moser R. The clinical and parasitological presentation of *P. falciparum* malaria in Uganda is unaffected by HIV infection. *Transactions of the Royal Society of Tropical Medicine and Hygiene* 84: 336–338 (1990)

Müller O, Moser R. HIV-1 disease in a Kampala Hospital. *The Lancet* 335: 236–237 (1990)

Müller O, Moser R, Guggenberger P, Alexander M. AIDS in Africa. *The New England Journal of Medicine* 12: 847–848 (1991)

Müller O, Quinones M, Cham K, Aikins M, Greenwood B. Detecting permethrin on treated bednets. *The Lancet* 344: 1699–1700 (1994)

Müller O, Van Hensbroek M, Jaffar S, Drakeley C, Okorie C, Joof D, Pinder M, Greenwood B. A randomized trial of chloroquine, amodiaquine, and pyrimethamine-sulfadoxine in Gambian children with uncomplicated malaria. *Tropical Medicine and International Health*. 1: 124–132 (1996)

Müller O, Cham K, Jaffar S, Greenwood B. The Gambian National Impregnated Bed net Programme – evaluation of the 1994 cost recovery trial. *Social Science and Medicine* 44: 1903–1909 (1997)

Müller O, Corrah T, Katabira E, Plummer F, Mabey D. Antiretroviral therapy in sub-Saharan Africa. *The Lancet* 351: 68 (1998)

Müller O, Garenne M. Childhood mortality in Africa. *The Lancet* 353: 673 (1999)

Müller O. History and State of Global Malaria Control. *Acta Leopoldina* 80, 313: 127–49 (2000)

Müller O, Becher H, Baltussen A, Ye Y, Diallo D, Konate M, Gbangou A, Kouyate B, Garenne M. Effect of zinc supplementation on malaria morbidity among Westafrican children: a randomized double-blind placebo-controlled trial. *BMJ* 322: 1567–1572 (2001)

Müller O, Ido K, Traoré C. Evaluation of a prototype long-lasting insecticide-treated mosquito net under field conditions in rural Burkina Faso. *Transactions of the Royal Society of Tropical Medicine and Hygiene* 96: 483–484 (2002)

Müller O, Traoré C, Kouyaté B, Becher H. Malaria morbidity, treatment seeking behaviour, and mortality in a cohort of young children in rural Burkina Faso. *Tropical Medicine and International Health* 8: 290–296 (2003)

Müller O, Jahn A. Expanding insecticide-treated mosquito net coverage in Africa: tradeoffs between public and commercial strategies. *Tropical Medicine & International Health* 8: 853–6 (2003)

Müller O. Malaria: Ein bedeutendes Entwicklungshindernis in Afrika. In: Gesundheit und Entwicklung in der Dritten Welt. Veröffentlichungen des Interdisziplinären Arbeitskreises Dritte Welt, Band 17, Seite 21–38, Johannes Gutenberg Universität Mainz (2004)

Müller O, Razum O, Traore C, Kouyate B. Community effectiveness of chloroquine and traditional remedies in the treatment of young children with falciparum malaria in rural Burkina Faso. *Malaria Journal* 3: 36 (2004)

Müller O, Krawinkel M. Review: Malnutrition and health in developing countries. *Journal of the Canadian Medical Association* 173: 279–86 (2005)

Müller O. Malaria. In: Razum, Zeeb & Laser (Eds.), Globalisierung – Gerechtigkeit – Gesundheit, Einführung in International Public Health (pp. 267–278). Verlag Hans Huber (2006)

Müller O, Becher H. Malnutrition and childhood mortality in developing countries. *The Lancet* 367: 1978 (2006)

Müller O, De Allegri M, Becher H, Tiendrebogo J, Beiersmann C, Ye M, Kouyate B, Sie A, Jahn A. Distribution systems of insecticide-treated bed nets for malaria control in rural Burkina Faso: cluster-randomized controlled trial. *PLoS One* e3182 (2008)

Müller O, Razum O. Primary Health Care: Die Neuauflage einer revolutionären Idee. *Deutsches Ärzteblatt* 105: A1841–43 (2008)

Müller O, Sié A, Meissner P, Schirmer RH, Kouyaté B. Artemisinin resistance on the Thai-Cambodian border. *The Lancet* 374: 1418–19 (2009a)

Müller O, Yé M, Louis V, Sié A. Malaria in sub-Saharan Africa. *The Lancet* 373: 122 (2009b)

Müller O, Jahn A. Chapter 16: Malnutrition and Maternal and Child Health. In: Ehiri (Ed), Maternal and Child Health (pp. 287–310). Springer US (2010)

Murray CJL, Frenk J, Evans T. The Global Campaign for the Health MDGs: challenges, opportunities, and the imperative of shared learning. *The Lancet* 370: 1018–21 (2007a)

Murray CJL, Laakso T, Shibuya K, Hill K, Lopez AD. Can we achieve MDG 4? New analysis of country trends and forecasts of under-5 mortality to 2015. *The Lancet* 370: 1040–54 (2007b)

Mushi AK, Schellenberg JRM, Mponda H, Lengeler C. Targeted subsidy for malaria control with treated nets using a discount voucher system in Tansania. *Health Policy and Planning* 18: 163–71 (2003)

Mutabingwa TK, Anthony D, Heller A, Hallett R, Ahmed J, Drakeley C, Greenwood BM, Whitty CJ. Amodiaquine alone, amodiaquine + sulfadoxine-pyrimethamine, amodiaquine + artesunate, and artemether lumefantrine for outpatient treatment of malaria in Tanzanian children: a four-arm randomised effectiveness trial. *The Lancet* 365: 1474–80 (2005)

Mwenesi HA. Social science research in malaria prevention, management and control in the last two decades: An overview. *Acta Tropica* 95: 292–97 (2005)

Nabarro D, Tayler E. The „roll back malaria" campaign. *Science* 280: 2067–2068 (1998)

Najera J. Malaria and the work of WHO. *Bulletin of the World Health Organization* 67: 229–243 (1989)

Najera J. Malaria control: achievements, problems and strategies. *Parassitologia* 43: 1–89 (2001)

Narasimhan V, Brown H, Pablos-Mendez A, Adams O, Dussault G, Elzinga G, Nordstrom A, Habte D, Jacobs M, Solimano G, Sewankambo N, Wibulpolprasert S, Evans T, Chen L. Responding to the global human resources crisis. *The Lancet* 363: 1469–72 (2004)

Ndugwa RP, Ramroth H, Müller O , Jasseh M, Sié A, Kouyaté B, Greenwood B, Becher H. Comparison of all-cause and a malaria-specific mortality from two West African countries with different malaria transmission patterns. *Malaria Journal* 7: 15 (2008)

Needham CA, Canning R. Global Disease Eradication. The race for the last child. *ASM Press*. Washington (2003)

Nevill C, Some E, Mungala V., Mutemi W, New L, Marsh K, Lengeler C, Snow R. Insecticide-treated bed nets reduce mortality and severe morbidity from malaria among children on the Kenyan coast. *Tropical Medicine & International Health* 1: 139–46 (1996)

Newman RD. Malaria control beyond 2010. *BMJ* 340: c2714 (2010)

Newton PN, Green MD, Fern'andez FM, Day NPJ, White NJ. Counterfeit anti-infective drugs. *The Lancet Infectious Diseases* 6:602–613 (2006a)

Newton PN, White NJ, Rozendaal JA, Green MD. Murder by fake drugs. *BMJ* 324:800–801 (2002)

N'Guessan R, Corbel V, Akogbeto M, Rowland M. Reduced efficacy of ITN and IRS for malaria control in pyrethroid resistance area, Benin. *Emerging Infectious Diseases* 13: 199–206 (2007)

Noedl H, Se Y, Schaecher K, Smith BL, Socheat D, Fukuda MM. Artemisinin Resistance in Cambodia 1 (ARC1) Study Consortium. Evidence of artemisinin-resistant malaria in western Cambodia. *The New England Journal of Medicine* 11;359:2619–20 (2008)

Noor AM, Metheu JJ, Tatem AJ, Hay SI, Snow RW. Insecticide-treated net coverage in Africa: mapping progress in 2000–07. *The Lancet* 373: 58–67 (2009)

Nosten F, Brasseur P. Combination therapy for malaria – the way forward? *Drugs* 62: 1315–29 (2002)

Nosten F, van Vugt M, Price R, Luxemburger C, Thway KL, Brockman A, McGready R, ter Kuile F, Looareesuwan S, White NJ. Effects of artesunate-mefloquine combination on incidence of Plasmodium falciparum malaria and mefloquine resistance in western Thailand: a prospective study. *The Lancet* 356: 297–302 (2000)

Nshakira N, Kristensen M, Ssali F, Whyte SR. Appropriate treatment of malaria? Use of antimalarial drugs for children's fevers in district medical units, drug shops and homes in eastern Uganda. *Tropical Medicine & International Health* 7: 309–316 (2002).

Nsimba SED, Warsame M, Tomson G, Massele A, Mbatiya Z. A household survey of source, availability, and use of antimalarials in a rural areas of Tanzania. *Drug Information Journal* 33:1025–32 (1999)

Nsungwa-Sabiiti J, Petedrson S, Pariyo G, Ogwal-Okeng J, Petzold MG, Tomson G. Home-based management of fever and malaria treatment practices in Uganda. *Transactions of the Royal Society of Tropical Medicine and Hygiene* 101: 1199–1207 (2007)

Nyarango PM, Gebremeskel T, Mebrahtu G, Mufunda J, Abdulmumini U, Ogbamariam A, Kosia A, Gebremichael A, Gunawardena D, Ghebrat Y, Okbaldet Y. A steep decline of malaria morbidity and mortality trends in Eritrea between 2000 and 2004: the effect of combination of control methods. *Malaria Journal* 5: 33 (2006)

Okie S. A new attack on malaria. *The New England Journal of Medicine* 358: 2425–28 (2008)

Okoye PN, Brooke BD, Koekemoer LL, Hunt RH, Coetzee M. Characterisation of DDT, pyrethroid and carbamate resistance in Anopheles funestus from Obuasi, Ghana. *Transactions of the Royal Society of Tropical Medicine and Hygiene* 102: 591–8 (2008)

Okrah J, Traoré C, Palé A, Sommerfeld J, Müller O. Community factors associated with malaria prevention by mosquito nets: an exploratory study in rural Burkina Faso. *Tropical Medicine & International Health* 7: 240–248 (2002)

Oliveira-Cruz V, Kurowski C, Mills A. Delivery of priority health services: searching for synergies within the vertical versus horizontal debate. *Journal of International Development* 15: 67–86 (2003)

Ollario P, Wells TNC. The global portfolio of new antimalarial medicines under development. *Clinical Pharmacology & Therapeutics* 85: 584–95 (2009)

Omaswa F: Human resources for global health: time for action is now. *The Lancet* 371: 625–6 (2008)

O'Meara WP, Bejon P, Mwangi TW, Okiro EA, Peshu N, Snow RW, Newton CR, Marsh K. Effect of a fall in malaria transmission on morbidity and mortality in Kilifi, Kenya. *The Lancet* 372: 1555–62 (2008)

O'Meara WP, Mangeni JN, Steketee R, Greenwood B. Changes in the burden of malaria in sub-Saharan Africa. *The Lancet Infectious Diseases* 10: 545–55 (2010)

Onori E, Beales P, Gilles H. From malaria eradication to malaria control: the past, the present and the future. In: Bruce-Chwatt`s Essential Malariology. Edited by Gilles and Warrell. Boston: *Little, Brown and Company* (1993a)

Onori E, Beales P, Gilles H. Rationale and technique of malaria control. In: Bruce-Chwatt`s Essential Malariology. Edited by Gilles and Warrell. Boston: *Little, Brown and Company* (1993b)

Ooms G, Van Damme W, Bakers BK, Zeitz P, Schrecker T. The ,diagonal' approach to Global Fund financing: a cure fort he broader malaise of health systems? *Globalization and Health* 4:6 (2008)

Orimadegun AE, Fawole O, Okereke JO, Akinbambi FO, Sodeinde O. Increasing burden of childhood severe malaria in a Nigerian tertiary hospital: implications for control. *Journal of Tropical Pediatrics* 53: 185–89 (2007)

Otten M, Aregawi M, Were W, Karema C, Medin A, Bekele W, Jima D, Gausi K, Komatsu R, Korenromp E, Low-Beer D, Grabowsky M. Initial evidence of reduction of malaria cases and deaths in Rwanda and Ethiopia due to rapid scale-up of malaria prevention and treatment. *Malaria Journal* 8: 14 (2009)

Ouedraogo A, Tiono AB, Diarra A, Nébié IO, Konaté AT, Sirima SB. The effects of a pre-season treatment with effective antimalarials on subsequent malaria morbidity in under five-year-old children living in high and seasonal malaria transmission area of Burkina Faso. *Tropical Medicine & International Health* 15: 1315–21 (2010)

Over M. The consequences of adult ill-health. In: the health of adults in the developing world. Editors: R. Feachem, T. Kjoellstrom, C. Murray, M. Over, M. Phillips. New York, *Oxford University Press* (1992)

Packard R. (2010) The Making of a Tropical Disease: A Short History of Malaria. *John Hopkins University Press*. ISBN 8-018-8712-3 (2008)

Pagnoni F, Convelbo N, Tiendrebeogo J, Cousens S, Esposito F: A community-based programme to provide promt and adequate treatment of presumptive malaria in children. *Transactions of the Royal Society of Tropical Medicine and Hygiene* 91:512–17 (1997)

Perkins MD, R Bell DR. Working without a blindfold: the critical role of diagnostics in malaria control *Malaria Journal*, 7 (supplement 1): 5 (2008)

Pfeiffer K, Some F, Müller O, Sie A, Kouyaté B, Haefeli WE, Zoungrana A, Gustafsson LL, Tomson G, Sauerborn R. Clinical diagnosis of malaria and the risk of chloroquine self-medication in rural health centres in Burkina Faso. *Tropical Medicine & International Health* 13: 418–426 (2008)

Phillips-Howard PA, Nahlen BL, Kolczak MS, Hightower AW, ter Kuile FO, Alaii JA, Gimnig JE, Arudo J, Vulule JM, Odhacha A, Kachur SP, Schoute E, Rosen DH, Sexton JD, Oloo AJ, Hawley WA. Efficacy of permethrin-treated bed nets in the prevention of mortality in young children in an area of high perennial malaria. *American Journal of Tropical Medicine and Hygiene* 68 (supplement): 23–29 (2003)

Pillay N. Right to health and the Universal Declaration of Human Rights. *The Lancet* 372: 2005–06 (2008)

Piola P, Fogg C, Bajunirwe F, Biraro S, Grandesso F, Ruzagira E, Babigumira J, Kigozi I, Kiguli J, Kyomuhendo J, Ferradini L, Taylor W, Checchi F, Guthmann JP. Supervised versus unsupervised intake of six-dose atremether-lumefantrine for treatment of acute, uncomplicated Plasmodium falciparum malaria in Mbarara, Uganda: a randomised trial. *The Lancet* 365: 1467–73 (2005)

Plowe CV. The evolution of drug-resistant malaria. *Transactions of the Royal Society of Tropical Medicine and Hygiene* 103: S11–14 (2009)

PMI. *www.fightingmalaria.gov, accessed 11.10.2010* (2010)

Poser CM, Bruyn GW An illustrated history of malaria. ISBN 1-85070-068-0. *The Parthenon Publishing Group*, London (1999)

Price RN, Nosten F, Luxemburger C, Ter-Kuile FO, Paiphun L, Luxemburger C, Chongsuphajaisiddhi T, White NJ, Nosten F, White NJ. Effects of artemisinin derivates on malaria transmissibility. *The Lancet* 347: 1654–58 (1996)

Protopopoff N, Van Bortel WV, Speybroeck N, Van Geertruyden JP, Baza D, D'Alessandro U, Coosemans M. Ranking Malaria Risk Factors to Guide Malaria Control Efforts in African Highlands. *PloS One* 11: 8022 (2009)

Radloff P, Philipps J, Nkeyi M, Hutchinson D, Kremsner P. Atovaquone plus proguanil for Plasmodium falciparum malaria. *The Lancet* 347: 1511–1514 (1996)

Ramroth H, Ndugwa RP, Müller O, Yé Y, Sie A, Kouyaté B, Becher H. Decreasing childhood mortality and increasing proportion of malaria deaths in rural Burkina Faso. *Global Health Action* 2 (2009)

Ranson H, Jensen B, Vulule JM, Wang X, Hemingway J, Collins FH. Identification of a point mutation in the volatge-gated sodium channel gene of Kenya *Anopheles gambiae* associated with resistance to DDT and pyrethroids. *Insect Molecular Biology* 95: 491–97 (2000)

Ranson H, N'Guessan R, Lines J, Moiroux N, Nkuni Z, Corbel V. Pyrethroid resistance in African anopheline mosquitoes: what are the implications for malaria control? *Trends in Parasitology* 26:1–8 (2010)

Ranson H, Abdallah H, Badolo A, Guelbeogo WM, Kerah-Hinzoumbe C, Yangalbe-Kalnone E, Sagnon N, Simard F, Coetzee M. Insecticide resistance in Anopheles gambiae: data from the first year of a multi-country study highlight the extent of the problem. *Malaria Journal* 8: 299 (2009)

Ratcliff A, Siswantoro H, Kenangalem E, Maristela R, Wuwung RM, Laihad F, Ebsworth EP, Anstey NM, Tjitra E, Price RN. Two fixed dose artemisinin combinations for drug-resistant falciparum and vivax malaria in Papua, Indonesia: an open-label randomised comparison. *The Lancet* 369: 757–65 (2007)

Raufu A. Influx of fake drugs to Nigeria worries health experts. *BMJ* 324:698 (2002)

Ray A. Malaria control, achivements, problems and prospects of eradication. *Journal of Communal Diseases* 9: 145–171 (1977)

RBM. The Global Malaria Action Plan. Roll Back Malaria Partnership, World Health Organisation, Geneva (2008)

Reich MR, Takemi K, Roberts MJ, Hsiao WC. Global action on health systems: a proposal for the Toyako G8 summit. *The Lancet* 371: 865–69 (2008)

Reuben R. Women and malaria – special risks and appropriate control strategy. *Social Science and Medicine* 37: 473–480 (1993)

Reyburn H, Mbakilwa H, Mwangi R, Mwerinde O, Olomi R, Drakeley C, Whitty CJ. *BMJ* 334: 403 (2007)

Ridley RG, Fletcher ER. Making a difference: 30 years of TDR. *Nature Reviews* 6: 401–07 (2008)

Rohde J, Cousens S, Chopra M, Tangcharoensathien V, Black R, Bhutta ZA, Lawn JE. 30 years after Alma-Ata: has primary health care worked in countries? *The Lancet* 372: 950–61 (2008)

Roca-Feltrer A, Carneiro I, Smith L, Armstrong Schellenberg JRM, Greenwood B, Schellenberg D. The age patterns of severe malaria syndromes in sub-Saharan Africa across a range of transmission intensities and seasonality settings. *Malaria Journal* 9:282 (2010)

Rogerson SJ, Carter R. Severe vivax malaria: newly recognised or rediscovered? *PLoS Medicine* 5: e136 (2008)

Rogier C, Ly AB, Tall A, Cisse´ B, Trape´ JF. Plasmodium falciparum malaria in Dielmo, a holoendemic area in Senegal: no influence of acquired immunity on initial symptomatology and severity of malaria attacks. *American Journal of Tropical Medicine and Hygiene* 60: 410–420 (1999)

Rozendaal J. Fake antimalaria drugs in Cambodia. *The Lancet* 357: 890 (2001)

Ruebush T, Kern, M., Campbell C, Oloo A. Self-treatment of malaria in a rural area of western Kenya. *Bulletin of the World Health Organization* 73: 229–236 (1995)

Sabot O, Cohen JM, Hsiang MS, Kahn JK, Basu S, Tang L, Zheng B, Gao Q, Zou L, Tatarsky A, Aboobakar S, Usas J, Barett S, Cohen JL, Jamison DT, Feachem RGA. Malaria Elimination Series IV: Costs and financial feasibility of malaria elimination. *The Lancet* 376: 1604–15 (2010)

Sachs JD. Achieving the Millenium Development Goals – The Case of Malaria. *The New England Journal of Medicine* 352: 115–17 (2005)

Sachs JD. The MDG decade: looking back and conditional optimism for 2015. *The Lancet* 376: 950–51 (2010)

Sachs G, Malaney P. The economic and social burden of malaria. *Nature* 415: 680–685 (2002)

Sadasivaiah S, Tozan Y, Breman JG. Dichlorodiphenyltrichloroethane (DDT) for Indoor Residual Spraying in Africa: How Can It Be Used for Malaria Control? *American Journal of Tropical Medicine and Hygiene* 77 (supplement 6): 249–263 (2007)

Sadiq S, Glasgow K, Drakeley C, Müller O, Greenwood B, Mabey D, Bailey R. Effects of azithromycin on malariometric indices in The Gambia. *The Lancet* 346: 881–882 (1995)

Samb B, Desai N, Nishtar S, Mendis S, Bekedam H, Wright A, Hsu J, Martiniuk A, Celletti F, Patel K, Adshead F, McKee M, Evans T, Alwan A, Etienne C. Prevention and management of chronic disease: a litmus test for health-systems strengthening in low-income and middle-income countries. *The Lancet* 376: 1785–97 (2010)

Sauerborn R, Nougtara A, Hien M, Diesfeld HJ. Seasonal variations of the household costs of illness in Burkina Faso. *Social Science and Medicine* 43: 281–290 (1996)

Sazawal S, Black RE, Ramsan M, Chwaya HB, Stoltzfus RJ, Dutta A, Dhingra U, Kabole I, Deb S, Othman MK, Kabole FM. Effects of routine prophylactic supplementation with iron and folic acid on admission to hospital and mortality in preschool children in a high malaria transmission setting: community-based, randomised, placebo-controlled trial. *The Lancet* 367: 133–143 (2006)

Schellenberg D, Menendez C, Kahigwa E, Aponte J, Vidal J, Tanner M, Mshinda H, Alonso P. Intermittent treatment for malaria and anaemia control at time of routine vaccinations in Tanzanian infants: a randomised, placebo-controlled trial. *The Lancet* 357: 1471–1477 (2001)

Schellenberg D, Menendez C, Aponte JJ, Kahigwa E, Tanner M, Mshinda H, Alonso P. Intermittent preventive antimalarial treatment for Tanzanian infants: follow-up to age 2 years of a randomised, placebo-controlled trial. *The Lancet* 365: 1481–1483 (2005)

Schirmer H, Coulibaly B, Stich A, Scheiwein M, Merkle H, Eubel J, Becker K, Becher H, Müller O, Zich T, Schiek W, Kouyaté B. Methylene blue as an antimalarial agent – past and future. *Redox Report* 8: 272–76 (2003)

Schultz L, Steketee R, Chitsulo L, Macheso A, Kazembe P, Wirima J. Evaluation of maternal practices, efficacy, and cost-effectiveness of alternative antimalarial regimens for use in pregnancy: chloroquine and sulphadoxine-pyrimethamine. *American Journal of Tropical Medicine and Hygiene* 55 (supplement): 87–94 (1996)

Schultz L, Steketee R, Macheso A, Kazembe P, Chitsulo L, Wirima J. The efficacy of antimalarial regimens containing sulphadoxine-pyrimethamine and/or chloroquine in preventing peripheral and placental falciparum infection among pregnant women in Malawi. *American Journal of Tropical Medicine and Hygiene* 51: 515–522 (1994)

Service M. The Anopheles vector. In: Bruce-Chwatt's Essential Malariology. Edited by Gilles and Warrell. Boston: *Little, Brown and Company* (1993)

Shah NK. Assessing strategy and equity in the elimination of malaria. *PLoS Medicine* 7: e1000312 (2010)

Shanks GD. For severe malaria, artesunate is the answer. *The Lancet* 376: 1621–22 (2010)

Shakoor O, Taylor RB, Behrens RH. Assessment of the incidence of substandard drugs in developing countries. *Tropical Medicine & International Health* 2: 839–845 (1997)

Sharma VP. Current scenario of malaria in India. *Parassitologia* 41: 349–53 (1999)

Sharp BL, Kleinschmidt I, Streat E, Maharaj R, Barnes KI, Durrheim DN, Ridl FC, Morris N, Seocharan I, Kunene S, La Grange JJP, Jotham D, Mthembu JD, Francois Maartens F, Carrin L, Martin CL, Barreto A. Seven years of regional malaria control collaboration – Mosambique, South Africa, and Swaziland. *American Journal of Tropical Medicine and Hygiene* 76: 42–47 (2007)

Shaukat AM, Breman JG, McKenzie FE. Using the entomological inoculation rate to assess the impact of vector control on malaria parasite transmission and elimination. *Malaria Journal* 2010, 9:122

Shiffman J. Has donor prioritization of HIV/AIDS displaced aid for other health issues? *Health Policy and Planning* 23: 95–100 (2008)

Shulman C, Dorman E, Talisuna A, Lowe, B, Nevill C, Snow R, Jilio H, Peshu N, Bulmer J, Graham S, Marsh K. A community randomized controlled trial of insecticide-treated bed nets for the prevention of malaria and anaemia among primigravid women on the Kenyan coast. *Tropical Medicine & International Health* 3: 197–204 (1998)

Shulman C, Dorman E, Cutts F, Kawuondo K, Bulmer J, Peshu N, Marsh K. Intermittent sulphadoxine-pyrimethamine to prevent severe anaemia secondary to malaria in pregnancy: a randomised placebo-controlled trial. *The Lancet* 353: 632–636 (1999)

Shulman CE, Marshall T, Dorman EK, Bulmer JN, Cutts F, Peshu N, Marsh K: Malaria in pregnancy: adverse effects on haemoglobin levels and birthweight in primigravidae. *Tropical Medicine & International Health* 6:770–778 (2001)

Sidhu ABS, Verdier-Pinard D, Fidock DA. Chloroquine resistance in *Plasmodium falciparum* malaria parasites conferred by pfcrt mutations. *Science* 298: 210–13 (2002)

Sie A, Louis VR, Gbangou A, Müller O, Niamba L, Stieglbauer G, Ye M, Kouyate B, Sauerborn R, Becher H. The Health and Demographic Surveillance System (HDSS) in Nouna, Burkina Faso, 1993–2007. *Global Health Action* 2010, 3: 5284

Simba DO, Kakoko DC, Warsame M, Premji Z, Gomes MF, Tomson G, Johansson E. Understanding caretakers' dilemma in deciding whether or not to adhere with referral advice after pre-referral treatment with rectal artesunate. *Malaria Journal* 9: 123 (2010)

Singh B, Kim Sung L, Matusop A, Radhakrishnan A, Shamsul SS, Cox-Singh J, Thomas A, Conway DJ. A large focus of naturally acquired *P. knowlesi* infections in human beings. *The Lancet* 363: 1017–24 (2004)

Sirima SB, Konaté A, Tiono AB, Convelbo N, Cousens S, Pagnoni F. Early treatment of childhood fevers with pre-packaged antimalarial drugs in the home reduces severe malaria morbidity in Burkina Faso. *Tropical Medicine & International Health* 8: 133–39 (2003)

Siva N. Tackling the booming trade in counterfeit drugs. *The Lancet* 376: 1725–26 (2010)

Skarbinski J, Ouma PO, Louise M. Causer LM, Kariuki SK, Barnwell JW, Alaii JA, de Oliveira AM, Zurovac D, Larson BA, Snow RW, Rowe AK, Laserson KF, Akhwale WS, Slutsker L, Hamel MJ. Effect of Malaria Rapid Diagnostic Tests on the Management of Uncomplicated Malaria with Artemether-Lumefantrine in Kenya: A Cluster Randomized Trial. *American Journal of Tropical Medicine and Hygiene* 80: 919–26 (2009)

Slutsker L, Bloland P, Steketee W, Wirima J, Heymann D, Breman J. Infant and second-year mortality in rural Malawi: causes and descriptive epidemiology. *American Journal of Tropical Medicine and Hygiene* 55 (supplement): 77–81 (1996)

Smith T, Schellenberg JA, Hayes RJ. Attributable fraction estimates and case definitions for malaria in endemic areas. *Statistics in Medicine* 13: 2345–2358 (1994)

Smith T, Hurt N, Teuscher T, Tanner M. Is fever a good sign for clinical malaria in surveys of epidemic communities? *American Journal of Tropical Medicine and Hygiene* 52:306–310 (1995)

Smith DL, Klein EY, McKenzie FE, Laxminarayan R. Prospective strategies to delay the evolution of anti-malarial drug resistance: weighing the uncertainty. *Malaria Journal* 9: 217 (2010)

Smithuis F, Kyaw MK, Phe O, Aye KZ, Htet L, Barends M, Lindegardh N, Singtoroj T, Ashley E, Lwin S, Stepniewska K, White NJ. Efficacy and effectiveness of dihydroartemisinin-piperaquine versus artesunate-mefloquine in falciparum malaria: an open-label randomised comparison. *The Lancet* 367:2075–85 (2006)

Snow RW, Armstrong JR, Forster D, Winstanley MT, Marsh VM, Newton CR, Waruiru C, Mwangi I, Winstanley PA, Marsh K. Childhood deaths in Africa: uses and limitations of verbal autopsies. *The Lancet* 340: 351–355 (1992)

Snow R, Marsh K. Will reducing *P. falciparum* transmission alter malaria mortality among African children? *Parasitology Today* 11: 188–190 (1995)

Snow R, Omumbo J, Lowe B, Molyneux C, Obiera J, Palmer A, Weber M, Pinder M, Nahlen B, Obonyo C, Newbold C, Gupta S, Marsh K. Relation between severe malaria morbidity in children and level of P. falciparum in Africa. *The Lancet* 349: 1650–54 (1997)

Snow RW, Nahlen B, Palmer A, Donnelly CA, Gupta S, Marsh K. Risk of severe malaria among African infants: direct evidence of clinical protection during early infancy. *Journal of Infectious Diseases* 177: 819 (1998)

Snow RW, Craig M, Deichmann U, Marsh K. Estimating mortality, morbidity and disability due to malaria among Africa's non-pregnant population. *Bulletin of the World Health Organization* 77: 624–40 (1999)

Snow RW, Guerra CA, Noor AM, Myint HY, Hay SI. The global distribution of clinical episodes of *Plasmodium falciparum* malaria. *Nature* 434: 214–17 (2005)

Snow RW, Guerra CA, Mutheu JJ, Hay SI. International Funding for Malaria Control in Relation to Populations at Risk of Stable *Plasmodium falciparum* transmission. *PLoS Medicine* 7: e142 (2008)

Snow RW, Marsh K. Malaria in Africa: progress and prospects in the decade since the Abuja Declaration. *The Lancet* 376: 137–39 (2010)

Somadjinga M, Lluberas M, Jobin WR. Difficulties in organising first indoor spray programme against malaria in Angola under the President's Malaria Initiative. *Bulletin of the World Health Organization* 87: 871–74 (2009)

South East Asian Quinine Artesunate Malaria Trial (SEAQUAMAT) group. Artesunate versus quinine for the treatment of severe falciparum malaria: a randomised trial. *The Lancet* 366: 717–25 (2005)

Specht S, Hoerauf A. Does helminth elimination promote or prevent malaria? *The Lancet* 369:446–7 (2007)

Spencer H, Kaseje D, Mosley W, Sempebwa E, Huong A, Roberts J. Impact on mortality and fertility of a community-based malaria control program in Saradidi, Kenya. *Annals of Tropical Medicine and Parasitology* 81 (supplement): 36–45 (1987)

Sridar D, Batniji R. Misfinancing global health: a case for transparency in disbursements and decision making. *The Lancet* 372: 1185–91 (2008)

Sridhar D. Improving aid for maternal, newborn, and child health. The Lancet 376: 1444–45 (2010)

Ssekabira U, Bukirwa H, Hopkins H, Namagembe A, Weaver MR, Sebuyira LM, Quick L, Staedke S, Yeka A, Kiggundu M, Schneider G, McAdam K, Wabwire-Mangen F, Dorsey G. Improved malaria case management after integrated team-based training of health care workers in Uganda. *American Journal Tropical Medicine and Hygiene* 79: 826–33 (2008)

Staedke SG, Mwebaza N, Kamya MR, Clark TD, Dorsey G, Rosenthal PJ, Whitty CJ. Home management of malaria with artemether-lumefantrine compared with standard care in urban Ugandan children: a randomised controlled trial. *The Lancet* 373: 1623–1631 (2009)

Steketee R, Nahlen B, Parise M, Menendez C. The burden of malaria in pregnancy in malaria-endemic areas. *American Journal of Tropical Medicine and Hygiene* 64(1,2):28–35 (2001)

Steketee RW, Wirima JJ, Bloland PB, Chilima B, Mermin JH, Chitsulo L, Breman JG. Impairment of a pregnant woman's acquired ability to limit *Plasmodium falciparum* by infection with human immunodeficiency virus type-1. *American Journal of Tropical Medicine and Hygiene* 55: 42–49 (1996)

Stern AM, Markel H. International efforts to control infectious diseases, 1851 to the present. *JAMA* 292: 1474–79 (2004)

Stratton L, O'Neill MS, Kruk ME, Bell ML. The persistent problem of malaria: Addressing the fundamental causes of a global killer. *Social Science & Medicine* 67: 854–62 (2008)

Sutherland CJ, Ord R, Dunyo S, Jawara M, Drakeley CJ, Alexander N, Coleman R, Pinder M, Walraven G, Targett GAT. Reduction of malaria transmission to *Anopheles* mosquitoes with a six-dose regimen of co-artemether. *PLoS Medicine* 2: e92 (2005)

Takken W, Knols BGJ. Malaria vector control: current and future strategies. *Trends in Parasitology* 25, 3: 101–04 (2008)

Talisuna AO, Bloland P, D'Alessandro U. History, dynamics, and public health importance of malaria parasite resistance. *Clinical Microbiology Reviews* 17 (1): 235–54 (2004)

Talisuna A, Grewal P, Rwakimari JB, Mukasa S, Jagoe G, Banerji J. Cost is killing patients: subsidising effective antimalarials. *The Lancet* 374:1224–26 (2009)

Tanner, M, Vlassoff C. Treatment-seeking behaviour for malaria: a typology based on endemicity and gender. *Social Science and Medicine* 46: 523–532 (1998)

Tanner M, de Savigny D. Malaria eradication back on the table. *Bulletin of the World Health Organization* 86: 82–83 (2008)

Targett GA, Greenwood BM. Malaria vaccines and their potential role in the elimination of Malaria. *Malaria Journal* 7: S10 (2008)

Tatem AJ, Smith DL, Gething PW, Kabaria CW, Snow RW, Hay SI. Malaria Elimination Series II: Ranking of elimination feasibility between malaria-endemic countries. *The Lancet* 376: 1579–91 (2010)

Teklehaimanot A, McCord GC, Sachs JD. Scaling up malaria control in Africa: an economic and epidemiological assessment. *American Journal of Tropical Medicine and Hygiene* 77: 138–44 (2007)

Ter Kuile FO, Terlouw DJ, Phillips-Howard PA, Hawley WA, Friedmann JF, Kariuki SK, Shi YP, Kolczak MS, Lal AA, Vulule JM, Nahlen BL. Reduction of malaria during pregnancy by permethrin-treated bed nets in an area of intense perennial malaria transmission in western Kenya. *American Journal of Tropical Medicine and Hygiene* 68 (supplement): 50–60 (2003)

Tipke M, Diallo S, Coulibaly B, Störzinger D, Hoppe-Tichy T, Sie A, Müller O. Substandard anti-malarial drugs in Burkina Faso. *Malaria Journal* 7: 95 (2008)

Tipke M, Louis V, Yé M, De Allegri M, Beiersmann C, Sié A, Müller O, Jahn A. Access to malaria treatment in young children of rural Burkina Faso. *Malaria Journal* 8:266 (2009)

Tipke M. Malaria treatment in rural Burkina Faso: Treatment-seeking behaviour, availability, prices, and quality of drugs. Doctoral Thesis, *Ruprecht-Karls-University Heidelberg* (2010)

Tjitra E, Anstey NM, Sugiarto P, Warikar N, Kenangalem E, Karyana M, Lampah DA, Price RN. Multidrug-resistant P. vivax associated with severe and fatal malaria: a prospective study in Papua, Indonesia. *PLoS Medicine* 5: e128 (2008)

Tozan Y, Klein EY, Darley S, Panicker R, Laxminarayan R, Breman JG. Prereferral rectal artesunate for severe childhood malaria: a cost-effectiveness analysis. The Lancet 376: early online publication, 30. November (2010)

Tran TH, Dolecek C, Pham PM, Nguyen TD, Nguyen TT, Le HT, Dong TH, Tran TT, Stepniewska K, White NJ, Farrar J. Dihydroartemisinin-piperaquine against multidrug-resistant Plasmodium falciparum malaria in Vietnam: randomised clinical trial. *The Lancet* 363:18–22 (2004)

Traoré C. The epidemiology of malaria in a holoendemic area of rural Burkina Faso. Doctoral Thesis, *Ruprecht-Karls-University Heidelberg* (2003)

Trape JF, Rogier C, Konate L, Diagne N, Bouganali H, Canque B, Legros F, Badji A, Ndiaye G, Ndiaye P, Brahimi K, Faye O, Druilhe P, Silva LP. The Dielmo Project: a longitudinal study of natural malaria infection and the mechanisms of protective immunity in a community living in a holoendemic area of Senegal. *American Journal of Tropical Medicine and Hygiene* 51 (2): 123–137 (1994)

Trape J, Rogier C. Combating malaria morbidity and mortality by reducing transmission. *Parasitology Today* 12: 236–240 (1996)

Trape J. The public health impact of chloroquine resistance in Africa. *American Journal of Tropical Medicine and Hygiene* 64: S12–S17 (2001)

Trigg P, Condrachine A. Malaria control in the 1990s. *Bulletin of the World Health Organization* 76: 11–16 (1998)

Tshefu AK, Gaye O, Kayentao K, Thompson R, Bhatt KM, Sesay SS, Bustos DG, Tjitra E, Bedu-Addo G, Borghini-Fuhrer I, Duparc S, Shin CS, Fleckenstein L. Pyronaridine-artesunate Study Team. Efficacy and safety of a fixed-dose oral combination of pyronaridine-artesunate compared with artemether-lumefantrine in children and adults with uncomplicated *Plasmodium falciparum* malaria: a randomised non-inferiority trial. *The Lancet* 375: 1457–67 (2010)

UNITAID. *www.unitaid.eu, accessed 12.10.2010* (2010)

Van Damme W, Kober K, Laga M. The real challenges for scaling up ART in SSA. *AIDS* 20: 653–56 (2006)

Verhoeff FH, Brabin BJ, Hart CA, Chimsuku L, Kazembe P, Broadhead RL. Increased prevalence of malaria in HIV-infected pregnant women and its implications for malaria control. *Tropical Medicine & International Health* 4: 5–12 (1999)

Verle P, Lieu,T, Kongs A, Van Der Stuyft P, Coosemans M. Control of malaria vectors: cost analysis in a province of northern Vietnam. *Tropical Medicine & International Health* 4: 139–145 (1999)

Victora CG, Hanson K, Bryce J, Vaughan P. Achieving universal coverage with health interventions. *The Lancet* 364: 1541–48 (2004)

Von Seidlein l, Bojang K, Jones P, Jaffar S, Pinder M, Obaro S, Doherty T, Haywood M, Snougou G, Gemperli P, Gathmann I, Royce C, McAdam K, Greenwood B. A randomized controlled trial of arthemeter/benflumetol, a new antimalarial, and pyrimethamine/sulfadoxine in the treatment of uncomplicated falciparum malaria in African children. *American Journal of Tropical Medicine and Hygiene* 58: 638–644 (1998)

Von Seidlein L, Walraven G, Milligan PJ, Alexander N, Manneh F, Deen JL, Coleman R, Jawara M, Lindsay SW, Drakeley C, De Martin S, Olliaro P,

Bennett S, Schim van der Loeff M, Okunoye K, Targett GA, McAdam KP, Doherty JF, Greenwood BM, Pinder M. The effect of mass administration of sulfadoxine-pyrimethamine combined with artesunate on malaria incidence: a double-blind, community-randomized, placebo-controlled trial in The Gambia. *Transactions of the Royal Society of Tropical Medicine and Hygiene* 97 (2): 217–25 (2003)

Von Seidlein L, Deen JL. Pre-referral rectal artesunate in severe malaria. *The Lancet* 373: 522–23 (2009)

Wakabi W. Big hurdles remain in Africa's fight against malaria. *The Lancet Infectious Diseases* 10: 10 (2010)

Wakilzadeh W. Die Rolle von Merozoite Surface Protein-1 (MSP-1-Antikörper im Schutz von Säuglingen vor Malaria tropica in einem Holoendemiegebiet von Burkina Faso. Doctoral Thesis, *Ruprecht-Karls-University Heidelberg,* Germany (2008)

Wang S, Lengeler C, Mtasiwa D, Mshana T, Manane L, Maro G, Tanner M. Rapid Urban Malaria Appraisal (RUMA) II: Epidemiology of urban malaria in Dar es Salaam (Tanzania) *Malaria Journal* 5:45 (2006)

Wang S, Lengeler C, Smith TA, Vounatsou P, Diadie DA, Pritroipa X, Convelbo N, Kientga M, Tanner M. Rapid urban malaria appraisal (RUMA) I: Epidemiology of urban malaria in Ouagadougou. *Malaria Journal* 4: 43 (2005)

Warrell, D. Treatment and prevention of malaria. In: Bruce-Chwatt`s Essential Malariology. Edited by Gilles and Warrell. Boston: *Little, Brown and Company* (1993)

Warrell D. Treatment of severe malaria. *Journal of the Royal Society of Medicine* 82 (supplement 17): 44–50 (1989)

Watson R. Donations to Global Fund fall short of targets set by major donors in March. *BMJ* 341: c5654 (2010)

Weaver LT, Beckerleg S. Is health a sustainable state? A village study in The Gambia. *The Lancet* 341: 1327–30 (1993)

Webb JR JLA. Humanity's burden: A global history of malaria. ISBN 978-0-521-85418-4. *Cambridge University Press*, Cambridge (2009a)

Webb JLA The long shadow of malaria interventions in tropical Africa. *The Lancet* 374: 1883–84 (2009b)

Webster PC. Uganda registers successes with child-health volunteers. *The Lancet* 374: 1735–36 (2009)

Wellings TE, Plowe CV. Chloroquine-resistant malaria. *The Journal of Infectious Diseases* 184: 770–76 (2001)

Wells TNC, Burrows JN, Baird JK. Targeting the hypnozoite reservoir of P. vivax: the hidden obstacle to malaria elimination. *Trends in Parasitology* 26: 145–51 (2010)

Wernsdorfer W. Epidemiology of drug resistance in malaria. *Acta Tropica* 56: 143–156 (1994)

White N. Antimalarial drug resistance: the pace quickens. *Journal of Antimicrobiology and Chemotherapy* 30: 571–585 (1992)

White N. The treatment of malaria. *The New England Journal of Medicine* 335: 800–806 (1996)

White N, Nosten F, Hien TT, Watkins W, Olliaro P. Averting a malaria disaster. *The Lancet* 353: 1965–67 (1999)

White NJ, Pongtavornpinyo W. The de novo selection of drug-resistant malaria parasites. *Proceedings of the Royal Society London* 270: 545–54 (2003)

White NJ. Review: Antimalarial drug resistance. *The Journal of Clinical Investigation* 113:1084–92 (2004)

White NJ. Intermittant presumptive treatment for malaria. *PLoS Medicine* 2: 28–33 (2005)

White NJ. Qinghaosu (artemisinin): The prize of success. *Science* 320: 330–34 (2008)

White NJ. Malaria. In: Cook & Zumla (Eds), Manson's Tropical Diseases (22. Edition). ISBN 0 70202 6409. *Saunders, Elsevier Science Limited* (2009)

Whitty CJM, Rowland M, Sanderson F, Mutabingwa TK. Malaria. *BMJ* 325: 1221–24 (2002)

Whitworth J, Morgan D, Quigley M, Smith A, Mayanja B, Eotu H, Omoding N, Okongo M, Malamba S, Ojwiya A. Effect of HIV-1 and increasing immunosuppression on malaria parasitaemia and clinical episodes in adults in rural Uganda: a cohort study. *The Lancet* 356: 1051–1056 (2000)

Whitworth JAG, Kokwaro G, Kinyanjui S, Snewin VA, Tanner M, Walport M, Sewankambo N. Strengthening capacity for health research in Africa. *The Lancet* 372: 1590–93 (2008)

WHO. Report on the malaria conference in equatorial Africa. *Technical Report Series* No. 38, World Health Organization Geneva (1951)

WHO/UNICEF. „Primary Health Care". Report of the International Conference on Primary Health Care. Alma Ata, USSR, September 6–12, Geneva (1978)

WHO Malaria Unit. Global malaria control. *Bulletin of the World Health Organization* 71: 281–284 (1993a)

WHO Technical Report Series 839. World Health Organisation Geneva (1993b)

WHO: World malaria situation in 1994. *Weekly Epidemiological Record* 72: 269–292 (1997)

WHO. The World Health Report 2000: health systems: improving performance. World Health Organization (2000)

WHO. Assessment and monitoring of antimalarial drug efficacy for the treatment of uncomplicated falciparum malaria. WHO/HTM/RBM/2003.50 (2003)

WHO. World Malaria Report 2005. WHO, Geneva (2005)

WHO. Global Malaria Programme. Indoor Residual Spraying. WHO/HTM/ MAL/2006.1112 (2006)

WHO. Model list of essential medicines. 15th edition. http://www.who.int/medicines/publications/essentialmedicines/en/index.html, accessed 13.05.2010 (2007)

WHO. Malaria RDT Performance I. ISBN 978 92 4 159807 1 (2008a)

WHO. World Malaria Report 2008. ISBN 978 92 4 156369 7, WHO, Geneva (2008b)

WHO. Malaria RDT Performance II. ISBN 978 92 4 159946 7 (2009a)

WHO. World Malaria Report 2009. ISBN 978 92 4 156390 1, WHO, Geneva (2009b)

WHO Maximizing Positive Synergies Collaborative Group. An assessment of interactions between global health initiatives and country health systems. *The Lancet* 373: 2137–69 (2009)

Wibulpolprasert S, Tangcharoensathien V, Kanchanachitra C: Three decades of primary health care: reviewing the past and defining the future. *Bulletin of the World Health Organization* 86: 3–4 (2008)

Williams HA, Jones COH. A critical review of behavioural issues related to malaria control in sub-Saharan Africa: what contributions have social scientists made? *Social Science & Medicine* 59: 501–23 (2004)

Wongsrichanalai C, Pickard AL, Wernsdorfer WH, Meshnick SR. Review: Epidemiology of drug-resistant malaria. *The Lancet Infectious Diseases* 2: 209–18 (2002)

Working Group 5 of the Commission on Macroeconomics and Health. Improving health outcomes of the poor. Geneva WHO (2002)

Yates A, N`Guessan R, Kaur H, Akogbéto M, Rowland M. Evaluation of KO-Tab 1-2-3®: a wash-resistant 'dip-it-yourself' insecticide formulation for long-lasting treatment of mosquito nets. *Malaria Journal* 4: 52 (2005)

Yates R. Universal health care and the removal of user fees. *The Lancet* 373: 2078–81 (2009)

Zarocostas J. Malaria treatment should begin with parasitological diagnosis where possible, says WHO. *BMJ* 340: c1402 (2010)

Zongo I, Dorsey G, Rouamba N, Tinto H, Dokomajilar C, Guiguemde RT, Rosenthal PJ, Ouedraogo JB. Artemether-lumefantrine versus amodiaquine plus sulfadoxine-pyrimethamine for uncomplicated falciparum malaria in Burkina Faso: a randomised non-inferiority trial. *The Lancet* 369: 491 (2007)

Zoungrana A, Coulibaly B, Sié A, Walter-Sack I, Mockenhaupt FP, Kouyaté B, Schirmer RH, Klose C, Mansmann U, Meissner P, Müller O. Safety and efficacy of methylene blue combined with artesunate or amodiaquine for uncomplicated falciparum malaria: a randomized controlled trial from Burkina Faso. *PLoS One* 3: e1630 (2008)

Zwang J, Ashley EA, Karema C, D'Alessandro U, Smithuis F, Dorsey G, Janssens B, Mayxay M, Newton P, Singhasivanon P, Stepniewska K, White NJ, Nosten F. Safety and Efficacy of Dihydroartemisinin-Piperaquine in Falciparum Malaria: A Prospective Multi-Centre Individual Patient Data Analysis. *PLoS One* 4: e6358 (2009)

# Challenges in Public Health

Im Zeitalter der Globalisierung lässt sich *Public Health* nicht mehr allein innerhalb von nationalen Grenzen betreiben: Pandemien, abnehmende Trinkwasservorräte und steigender Tabakkonsum sind nur einige Beispiele für eine Vielzahl von neuen Herausforderungen, die einen weiter reichenden, internationalen Blick erfordern. Zusätzlich trägt eine einseitig an Wirtschaftsinteressen orientierte Globalisierung zu der weltweit zunehmenden gesundheitlichen Ungleichheit bei. Die Globalisierung eröffnet andererseits aber neue Wege, auch über Staatsgrenzen und große Entfernungen hinweg Wissen und Erfahrungen auszutauschen und gemeinschaftlich zu handeln. Kernpunkte für *Public Health* sind dabei die international vergleichende Analyse von Gesundheitsproblemen und möglichen Lösungsansätzen sowie die wissenschaftlich basierte und gerechte Ausgestaltung von Gesundheitssystemen. Hierzu möchte die Buchreihe *Challenges in Public Health* einen Beitrag leisten.

In times of globalisation, Public Health can no longer be practiced within national borders alone. Pandemics, diminishing drinking water supplies and increasing tobacco consumption are examples of the many new challenges that require a cross-border, international approach. In addition, a globalisation that is narrowly focused on economic interests contributes to growing health inequalities worldwide. At the same time, globalisation offers new opportunities to exchange knowledge and experiences and to collaborate across national borders. Key issues for Public Health are an international comparison of health problems and of possible strategies to solve them, as well as an evidence-based and equitable development of health systems. The book series *Challenges in Public Health* aims to contribute to this endeavour.

# Medizin in Entwicklungsländern

## Herausgegeben von Prof. Hans Jochen Diesfeld

Band 18 Gerhard Heller: Krankheitskonzepte und Krankheitssymptome. Eine empirische Untersuchung bei den Tamang von Cautara/Nepal zur Frage der kulturspezifischen Prägung von Krankheitserleben. 1985.

Band 19 Hans-Jochen Diesfeld / Sigrid Wolter (Hrsg.): Medizin in Entwicklungsländern. Handbuch zur praxisorientierten Vorbereitung für medizinische Entwicklungshelfer. 5. neubearbeitete Auflage. 1989.

Band 20 Verena Kücholl: Soziokulturelle Wege des Heilens. Eine ethnomedizinische Analyse und Interpretation des Samkhya und der Heiltradition der Navajo. 1985.

Band 21 Frank-Peter Schelp (Ed.): Health Problems in Asia and in the Federal Republic of Germany. How to solve them? Proceedings of a seminar on "Techniques and Problems of Intervention Trials in Developing and Developed Countries". 1985.

Band 22 Rolf Heinmüller, Winfried Kern: Primäre Gesundheitsversorgung im südwestlichen Sudan. Eine Feldforschung bei den südsudanesischen Azande zur Evaluierung der Einflüsse des 'Primary Health Care'-Programms auf gesundheitliche Lage und allgemeine Lebensbedingungen. Detailed English Summary. 1987.

Band 23 Andreas Hahold/Axel Kroeger: Krankheitsbewältigung im Andenhochland Perus. Ergebnisse einer Bevölkerungsbefragung. 1986.

Band 24 Georg Kamm / Peter Witton / Hatibu Lweno: Anaesthesia Notebook for Medical Auxilaries. With special Reference to Anaesthesia Practice in Developing Countries. 1989.

Band 25 Alice S. Kuhn: Heiler und ihre Patienten auf dem Dach der Welt. Ladakh aus ethnomedizinischer Sicht. 1988.

Band 26 Wolfgang Bichmann: Community Involvement in Nepal's Health System. A case study of district health services management and the Community Health Leader scheme in Kaski district. 1989.

Band 27 M. Luisa Vázquez / Renate Lipowsky / Axel Kroeger: Malaria und kutane Leishmaniase in Kolumbien. Vorkommen, Volkskonzepte und traditionelle Behandlungsformen. 1989.

Band 28 Heinrich Berg / Axel Kroeger / Carmen Perez-Samaniego / Fernando Malo: Kranke Menschen – krankes Gesundheitswesen? Eine epidemiologische Untersuchung in Nord-Mexiko. 1989.

Band 29 Emmie Ho-Tsui / Margit Urhahn: Medizin und Gesundheitsforschung in Entwicklungsländern. Bibliographie des Instituts für Tropenhygiene 1984-1988. 1991.

Band 30 Thomas Lux: Gespräche mit afrikanischen Krankenpflegern und Heilern. Bilder von Krankheit im Mikrokosmos von Malanville(Benin), 1991.

Band 31 Christopher Knauth: Arzneimittelgebrauch armer Bevölkerungsschichten in städtischen Elendsvierteln Perus. Möglichkeiten und Grenzen der Gesundheitserziehung zum rationalen Arzneimittelgebrauch. 1991.

Band 32 Erhard Hinz: Geomedizinische und biogeographische Aspekte der Krankheitsverbreitung und Gesundheitsversorgung in Industrie- und Entwicklungsländern. 1991.

Band 33 Klaus Hoffmann: Psychiatrie in Afrika. Eine Einführung für Entwicklungshelfer. 1992.

Band 34 Dorothea Sich / Hans Jochen Diesfeld / Angelika Deigner / Monika Habermann (Hrsg.): Medizin und Kultur. Eine Propädeutik für Studierende der Medizin und der Ethnologie mit 4 Seminaren in Kulturvergleichender Medizinischer Anthropologie (KMA). 1993. 2., unveränd. Aufl. 1995.

Band 35 Annette Wiemann-Michaels: Die verhexte Speise. Eine ethnopsychosomatische Studie über das Depressive Syndrom in Nepal. 1994.

Band 36 Christine Loytved: Hebammen in Ozeanien zwischen traditioneller und westlicher Medizin. Weiterbildung traditioneller Hebammen in Westsamoa und Tonga. 1994.

Band 37 Andrea Materlik: Medizinisch-anthropologische Aspekte von Lepra im Amazonas und ihre Bedeutung für die Gesundheitserziehung. 1994.

Band 38 Oliver Razum: Improving Service Quality through Action Research, as applied in the Expanded Programme on Immunization (EPI). 1994.

Band 39 Ulrich Schramm: Einflußfaktoren auf die Akzeptanz von baulichen Anlagen der ländlichen Gesundheitseinheiten in Ägypten. Fallstudie am Beispiel der staatlichen Einheit in Zebeda unter Verwendung der Post-Occupancy Evaluation. 1995.

Band 40 Rainer Sauerborn / Adrien Nougtara / Hans Jochen Diesfeld (Eds.): Recherche sur les systèmes de santé: Le cas de la zone médicale de Solenzo, Burkina Faso. Auteurs: Rainer Sauerborn, Adrien Nougtara, Hans Jochen Diesfeld, Gaston Sorgho, Joseph Bidiga, Lougousse Tiébélessé, Eric Latimer, Roberto Sallier de La Tour, Uwe Brinkmann, Don Shepard. 1995.

Band 41 Rainer Sauerborn / Adrien Nougtara / Hans Jochen Diesfeld (Eds.): Les Côuts Economiques de la Maladie pour les Ménages au Milieu Rural du Burkina Faso. Avec des contributions de Rainer Sauerborn, Adrien Nougtara, Maurice Hien, Issouf Ibrango, Matthias Borchert, Justus Benzler, Eberhard Koob, Hans Jochen Diesfeld. 1996.

Band 42 Erhard Hinz: Helminthiasen des Menschen in Thailand. 1996.

Band 43 Matthias Perleth: Historical Aspects of American Trypanosomiasis (Chagas' Disease). 1997.

Band 44 Christiane Fischer: Über die Effektivität der Dorfgesundheitsarbeiterinnen innerhalb der Nichtregierungsorganisation ACCORD in Tamil Nadu/Südindien. Aktionsforschung im Rahmen der Gesundheitssystemforschung. 1998.

Band 45 Maureen Dar lang: Assessment of antenatal and obstetric care services in a rural district of Nepal. 1999.

Band 46 Julia Katzan: sòi mendan – Die Sache mit dem Wasser... Eine medizinethnologische Untersuchung zum Zusammenhang von Wasser und Krankheit aus indigener Sicht. 2001.

Band 47 Catharina Will: Malaria-Selbstmedikation mit Chloroquin In einem hyperendemischen Gebiet (Mali). 2001.

Band 48 Ansgar Gerhardus: Entscheidungsprozesse im Gesundheitssektor. Der Beitrag der Theorie der politischen Ökonomie. 2001.

Band 49 Sylvie Schuster: Der Schwangerschaftsabbruch im Grasland Kameruns. Medizin, Kultur und Praxis. 2004.

Band 50 Sascha Klotzbücher: Das ländliche Gesundheitswesen der VR China. Strukturen – Akteure – Dynamik. 2006.

### Challenges in Public Health

Editor: Prof. Dr. Oliver Razum

Band 51 Ulrich Ronellenfitsch: Cardiovascular Mortality among Ethnic German Immigrants from the Former Soviet Union. 2007.

Band 52 Manuela De Allegri: To Enrol or not to Enrol in Community Health Insurance. Case Study from Burkina Faso. 2007.

Band 53 Catherine Kyobutungi: Ethnic German Immigrants from the Former Soviet Union: Mortality from External Causes and Cancers. 2008.

Band 54 Maren Bredehorst: Information Systems for the Rehabilitation of Landmine Survivors. 2007.

Band 55 Sven Voigtländer / Gabriele Berg-Beckhoff / Oliver Razum: Gesundheitliche Ungleichheit. Der Beitrag kontextueller Merkmale. 2008.

Band 56 Oliver Razum / Jürgen Breckenkamp / Pitt Reitmaier (Hrsg.): Kindergesundheit in Entwicklungsländern. 2008.

Band 57 Steffen Fleßa: Costing of Health Care Services in Developing Countries. A Prerequisite for Affordability, Sustainability and Efficiency. 2009.

Band 58 Patrick Brzoska / Oliver Razum: Validity Issues in Quantitative Migrant Health Research. The Example of Illness Perceptions. 2010.

Band 59 Oliver Razum / Anna Reeske / Jacob Spallek (Hrsg.): Gesundheit von Schwangeren und Säuglingen mit Migrationshintergrund. 2011.

Band 60 Olaf Müller: Malaria in Africa. Challenges for Control and Elimination in the 21st Century. 2011.

www.peterlang.de